ETHICS
A Case Study from Fluency

ETHICS
A Case Study from Fluency

Edited by
Robert Goldfarb, Ph.D.

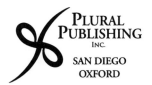

PLURAL
PUBLISHING
INC.

SAN DIEGO
OXFORD

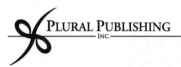

PLURAL PUBLISHING
INC.

5521 Ruffin Road
San Diego, CA 92123

e-mail: info@pluralpublishing.com
Web site: http://www.pluralpublishing.com

49 Bath Street
Abington, Oxfordshire OX14 1EA
United Kingdom

RC
424
.E79
2006
c.2

Copyright © by Plural Publishing, Inc. 2006

Typeset in 11/13 Palatino by Flanagan's Publishing Services, Inc.
Printed in the United States of America by McNaughton and
Gunn

For permission to use material from this text, contact us by
Telephone: (866) 758-7251
Fax: (888) 758-7255
e-mail: permissions@pluralpublishing.com

ISBN-13: 978-1-59756-010-8
ISBN-10: 1-59756-010-3
Library of Congress Control Number: 2005908653

CONTENTS

CONTRIBUTORS

Oliver Bloodstein, Ph.D.
Chapter 3

Dr. Bloodstein is Professor Emeritus of Speech at Brooklyn College of the City University of New York. An Honoree of the American Speech-Language-Hearing Association and the New York State Speech-Language Hearing Association, he is the author of *A Handbook on Stuttering; Stuttering: The Search for a Cause and Cure; Speech Pathology: An Introduction*, and numerous journal articles and research reports on stuttering.

Elizabeth Galletta, Ph.D.
Chapter 5

Dr. Galletta is an Associate Professor in the Communication Disorders Department at Mercy College where she teaches an undergraduate course in Organic Communication Disorders and graduate courses in Adult Language Disorders, Research Methods, and Fluency Disorders. She has mentored several graduate students' research projects in a variety of areas, including the area of second-language speech learning. She is a member of the Bilingualism Research Group at the Graduate Center of the City University of New York.

Robert Goldfarb, Ph.D.
Chapters 2 and 8

Dr. Goldfarb is Professor and Graduate Program Director of Communication Sciences and Disorders at Adelphi University, and Emeritus Professor of Speech and Hearing Sciences at Lehman College and the Graduate Center of CUNY. He is the author of numerous journal articles and book chapters on adult neurogenic communication disorders and coauthor of *Techniques for Aphasia Rehabilitation Generating Effective Treatment (TARGET)*, and *The Stocker Probe for Fluency and Language.* He has received the Distinguished Achievement Award from the New York State

Speech-Language-Hearing Association and the Professional Achievement Award from the New York City Speech-Language-Hearing Association, and is a member of the Academy of Aphasia.

Katherine S. Harris, Ph.D.
Chapter 7

Dr. Harris graduated from Radcliffe College and received a doctorate in experimental psychology from Harvard University. She joined the research staff of Haskins Laboratories in 1952 and is still affiliated there. She is Distinguished Professor Emerita in the Ph.D. Program in Speech and Hearing Sciences at the Graduate Center of the City University of New York. From 1975 to 1997 she was Principal Investigator for various grants, program projects, and review committees of the National Institutes of Health. She has published numerous papers and a textbook, *Speech Science Primer*, now in its fourth edition, coauthored with Gloria Borden and Lawrence Raphael. She is a fellow of the American Academy for the Advancement of Science, the American Speech-Language-Hearing Association, and the Acoustical Society of America. She has received the Honors of ASHA, and the Silver Medal in Speech Communication and the Rossing Medal for Education in Acoustics from the ASA.

Nicholas Johnson, LL.B.
Chapter 9

Dr. Johnson graduated from the University of Texas (Austin) with a B.A. in 1956 and an LL.B in 1958. He now teaches at the University of Iowa College of Law and formerly served as codirector of the university's Institute for Health, Behavior and Environmental Policy. He is perhaps best known as an FCC Commissioner (1966-1973) and author of *How to Talk Back to Your Television Set* (1970). A Web site with his writings and additional information is available at http://www.nicholasjohnson.org. He is the son of the Tudor study's supervisor, Dr. Wendell Johnson.

Loraine K. Obler, Ph.D.
Chapter 5

Dr. Obler is Distinguished Professor in the Program in Speech and Hearing Sciences of the Graduate Center of the City University of New York, with a joint appointment in Linguistics. Her publications include *The Bilingual Brain: Neuropsychological and Neurolinguistics of Bilingualism* (1978, with Martin Albert), *Agrammatism: A Cross-Language Narrative Sourcebook* (1990, edited with Lise Menn), and *Language and the Brain* (1999, with Kris Gjerlow). She has initiated colloquia on such ethical issues as plagiarism and authorship for doctoral students and faculty at the Graduate Center.

Gretchen Reynolds
Chapter 1

Ms. Reynolds writes about medicine, science, and other topics for *The New York Times Magazine, O: The Oprah Magazine, Popular Science, National Geographic Adventure*, and other publications. Part of a team that won a 2003 National Magazine Award for service writing, she lives in Santa Fe, New Mexico.

Barbara T. Schmidt, Ph.D.
Chapter 5

Dr. Schmidt is an Associate Professor and Program Director in the Speech-Language Pathology Program in the Communication Arts and Sciences Department at Molloy College. She teaches a variety of courses, including Psycholinguistic Models of Reading and Disorders of Communication. She has extensive clinical experience with adults who have acquired neurogenic disorders. Her research interest is in the cognitive-linguistic mechanisms of skilled reading. Of particular interest, are the cognitive mechanisms that enable compensatory reading strategies in individuals with persistently poor phonological awareness and acquired brain damage.

Richard G. Schwartz, Ph.D.
Chapter 6

Dr. Schwartz is Presidential Professor in the Ph.D. Program in Speech and Hearing Sciences and Chair of the Committee for the Protection of Human Subjects, the Graduate Center of the City University of New York. He attended McGill University, received his M.S. in Speech Pathology from the University of South Florida in 1974, and his Ph.D. in Speech Pathology and

Developmental Psychology from the University of Memphis (formerly Memphis State University) in 1978. Since 1978, Dr. Schwartz has held academic appointments at the University of Pittsburgh, Purdue University, The Graduate Center of the City of New York, Tel Aviv University, Weill Medical College of Cornell University and is currently a Visiting Professor of Otolaryngology at the Albert Einstein College of Medicine. Dr. Schwartz has published extensively on speech and language disorders in children in peer-reviewed scientific journals, contributed numerous chapters in academic textbooks and monographs, and has served as the editor of the *Journal of Speech, Language and Hearing Research*. He is the editor of the forthcoming *Handbook of Child Language Disorders* to be published by Psychology Press. Dr. Schwartz' research has been supported by grants from the National Institute on Deafness and Other Communication Disorders of the National Institutes of Health since 1979. He has served as the chair/organizer of numerous national and international conferences.

Ehud Yairi, Ph.D., CCC-SLP
Chapter 4

Dr. Yairi received his B.A. degree from Tel Aviv University, Israel, in Psychology and African Studies, and his M.A. and Ph.D. degrees in Speech-Language Pathology and Audiology from the University of Iowa. Currently he is a Professor Emeritus, Department of Speech and Hearing Science at the University of Illinois at Champaign-Urbana and is also affiliated with the Department of Communication Disorders, Tel Aviv University. For more than 35 years his research, much of it supported by the National Institutes of Health, has centered on many aspects of the onset and development of early childhood stuttering, including speech characteristics, environmental factors, and genetics. Among other indications of recognition, Yairi is the recipient of the *Malcolm Fraser Award* for excellence in the field of stuttering, the *Researcher Award of Distinction* from the International Fluency Association, and the highest award of the American Speech-Language-Hearing Association—the Honors of the Association.

INTRODUCTION

Mary Tudor, a graduate student at the University of Iowa, supervised by Wendell Johnson, conducted a study in 1939 to test Johnson's diagnosogenic theory of stuttering. The theory states the following:

1. The kind of speech shown by individuals who stutter at the onset of stuttering is not distinguishable from normal disfluency.

2. The diagnosis of stuttering is made by a lay person, usually a parent, which explains why stuttering runs in families.

3. Once the diagnosis is made, the child experiences disfluencies as speech failures, and begins avoidance and escape behaviors characteristic of stuttering.

Tudor and Johnson examined the effect of verbal labeling on the frequency of disfluency in both stuttering and fluent children, drawn from an orphanage in Davenport, Iowa. That they were allegedly able to induce stuttering in normally fluent children supported the hypothesis and raised serious ethical concerns, which have been recently reported widely in the media.

It is tempting and dangerous in a book dealing with ethics to seize the moral high ground. Cicero warns us about the dangers of hubris: "Why, upon the very books in which they bid us scorn ambition philosophers inscribe their names" (Collins, 2005). That said, we will be looking in detail about Wendell Johnson's diagnosogenic or semantogenic theory, which most of us learned in our undergraduate study. We are about to begin a critical review not only of the Tudor study, which is, after all, no more or less than a 66-year-old masters thesis, but also of ethics in scientific research. Before we start acting as critics, here is what has been said about them.

Lord Byron, in *English Bards and Scotch Reviewers* (part 1, line 75) is certainly no friend of critics. On the other hand, his comments about a woman would likely prompt a fairly strong critical reaction.

> As soon
> Seek roses in December, ice in June;
> Hope constancy in wind, or corn in chaff;
> Believe a woman or an epitaph,
> Or any other thing that's false, before
> You trust in critics.

Coleridge reminds us of the old saw, "Those who can do; those who can't teach." To which Woody Allen adds in his movie, *Annie Hall*, "Those who can't teach, teach gym." And Coleridge, in *Lectures on Shakespeare and Milton* (p. 36) says, in effect, "Those who can't teach gym become critics."

> Reviewers are usually people who would have been poets, historians, biographers, etc., if they could; they have tried their talents at one or at the other, and have failed; therefore they turn critics.

Finally, a favorite comment about critics comes from Isaac Asimov (1996) who, characteristically, considers them to be some alien race.

> His [Robert Frost's] poetry seems to please the critics, and because it is plain-spoken, rhymes and scans, it pleases human beings as well.

Before the events of September 11 overwhelmed everything else, the spring and summer of 2001 was a time for lively debate on ethics in communication disorders. There were several aspects of the debate that were remarkable:

1. It involved a masters thesis completed by Mary Tudor in 1939.

2. It involved the University of Iowa, where the profession of speech-language pathology in the United States began in the 1920s.

3. It involved the eminent Professor Wendell Johnson, who had died in1965.

As I followed the story, my initial reaction of surprise yielded to anger, then to doubt. The surprise was that Johnson, who was not only a founder of our profession, but one of its heroes, could be singled out for opprobrium based on unethical research. Anger followed the apology by the president of ASHA, on behalf of the Association, for the ethical lapses of a study done 62 years earlier. I felt it was inappropriate for the ASHA official to speak for more than one hundred thousand professionals, who could make their own decisions about the credibility of the accusation against Tudor and Johnson. Finally, there was the nagging doubt that the accusation was not completely without merit, as so many people in journalism, academe, and our national association joined in the rhetoric and hand-wringing.

The publication of an article by Ambrose and Yairi in 2002 was most welcome. In a critical review of what was called the Tudor study, the authors concluded that the data did not support the conclusion that labeling speech as stuttering induced the disorder in young children, and that Johnson's diagnosogenic theory was not supported. The time seemed right for a scholarly consideration of the substance of the debate. Was the Tudor study a small masters thesis whose hypotheses were not confirmed or was it, as the tabloids claimed, "The Monster Study," comparable to the Tuskegee syphilis study and Nazi "science"?

In my position at the time as Executive Officer of the Ph.D. Program in Speech and Hearing Sciences at the Graduate Center of CUNY, the nation's largest Ph.D. program, I determined to invite some of the major influences in the areas of stuttering and research to participate in a Symposium on Ethics and the Tudor Study. To my surprise and delight, everyone who was asked accepted the invitation. Among the participants were the following, in alphabetical order:

Oliver Bloodstein, Ph.D., Professor Emeritus, Brooklyn College of CUNY and ASHA Honoree, who was Wendell Johnson's most famous student and is considered by many to be the world's foremost living authority on stuttering.

Katherine S. Harris, Ph.D., Distinguished Professor Emerita at the Graduate Center of CUNY and ASHA Honoree, who was Principal Investigator of program project grants at Haskins Laboratories for 27 years, and was directly involved in much of the physiological research on stuttering.

Nicholas Johnson, LL.B., former FCC Commissioner and co-director of the University of Iowa Institute for Health, Behavior and Environmental Policy, current faculty member at the University of Iowa College of Law, and, not incidentally, Wendell Johnson's son.

Loraine K. Obler, Ph.D., Distinguished Professor of Linguistics and Speech and Hearing Sciences, Graduate Center of CUNY, and formerly that institution's Ombuds Officer.

Richard G. Schwartz, Ph.D., Presidential Professor of Speech and Hearing Sciences, Graduate Center of CUNY, ASHA Fellow, and Chair of the Institutional Review Board.

Ehud Yairi Ph.D., Professor of Communication Sciences and Disorders at the University of Illinois and ASHA Honoree, who has been Principal Investigator on major grants from the National Institute for Deafness and other Communication Disorders on the genetics of stuttering.

The Symposium on Ethics and the Tudor Study was held at the Graduate Center of CUNY on December 22, 2002. Shortly thereafter, I exchanged telephone calls and e-mail messages with Gretchen Reynolds, a frequent freelance contributor to *The New York Times*, who was preparing a long article on Wendell Johnson and the Tudor study for inclusion in a special Sunday *Times Magazine* dealing with health concerns. The article was published on March 16, 2003, and is reprinted here with permission of Ms. Reynolds and *The New York Times*.

The term "stutterers" does not appear in this volume, except when it is part of a direct quotation. The term "individual who stutters" or "person who stutters" is used instead. Although a person should obviously be known by more than a disability, it is somewhat better than being identified *as* the disability. It is also consistent with the position taken by ASHA a quarter century ago with regard to aphasia. Having been asked to write a chapter for the first edition of Chapey's (2001) well-known book on aphasia, first published in 1981, I received a Contributor Agreement in 1980 for a book to be called *Language Intervention Strategies for the Adult Aphasic*. After ASHA determined that "aphasic" should be used only as an adjective, and not as a noun, a new Contributor Agreement was sent, for the book entitled, *Language Intervention Strategies in Adult Aphasia*.

Political correctness of language can sometimes go too far. When Bloodstein was my teacher, he was preparing the first edition of his famous *Handbook on Stuttering*, now in its fifth edition (1995). The book, which cost two dollars then, was published by the National Easter Seal Society for Crippled Children and Adults. Most people would now recoil at the use of "crippled" to describe people afflicted with polio. Most, but not my brother-in-law, who has lived with polio since age 2. Mike does not want to be called "physically challenged," because, to him, a staircase is not a challenge but an impossibility.

As the Tudor study was a graduate thesis, the term "masters" degree was selected for uniformity. Alternate punctuation (master's, masters') and capitalization (Master's, Masters') appeared in manuscripts of contributing authors and were changed. On the other hand, I did not ask authors to restrict or include the first person singular or plural. Some were comfortable using "I" and "we" and some were not. I beg the reader's indulgence in permitting the authors to speak in their preferred voices.

There are many people to thank. The Stuttering Foundation provided financial support for the Symposium, and the two doctoral students who participated were Malcolm Fraser Fellows. *The New York Times*, The Speech Bin, and ASHA permitted the use of previously published material. Loretta Walker, Assistant Program Officer for Speech and Hearing Sciences at the Graduate Center, arranged many of the details associated with the Symposium. Taro Alexander brought his magnificent Our Time Theatre Company, a theatrical company for people who stutter, to perform in the evening after the Symposium.

Professor Florence Myers edited the editor, reviewing and improving my contributions to this volume. My graduate student research assistants at Adelphi University, especially Danielle Lavi and Nellyzita Offoha, helped in contacting authors, retyping manuscripts, and proofreading. The Adelphi Faculty Center for Professional Excellence provided assistance and equipment for preparing and updating figures and drawings. Mark Kalish, of Moss & Kalish, PLLC, provided guidance and references in my research on power of attorney. Sadanand Singh, Sandy Doyle, and Lauren Duffy of Plural Press were helpful, wise, and encouraging throughout the project. Most significant are Shelley and Elizabeth Goldfarb, whose contributions to my life cannot be measured in words.

References

Ambrose, N. G., & Yairi, E. (2002). The Tudor study: Data and ethics. *American Journal of Speech-Language Pathology, 11,* 190–203.

Asimov, I. (1996). *Magic* (p. 191). New York: HarperPrism.

Bloodstein, O. (1995). *A handbook on stuttering* (5th ed.). San Diego: Singular Publishing Group.

Chapey, R. (Ed.). (2001). *Language intervention strategies in aphasia and related neurogenic communication disorders* (4th ed.). Philadelphia: Lippincott Williams & Wilkins.

Collins, W. L. (2005). *The project Gutenberg ebook of Cicero.* Available from: www.gutenberg.org

THE STUTTERING DOCTOR'S "MONSTER STUDY"*

Gretchen Reynolds

Wendell Johnson was a tall, knobby 20-year-old farm boy when he arrived at the University of Iowa in Iowa City to study English in 1926. The class president and valedictorian of his tiny high school in Roxbury, Kansas, Johnson was engaging, "quite a clown" in the estimation of the folks back home. He also stuttered grotesquely, often rendered speechless by the impediment. His inability to express himself nudged him toward writing and literature, and he developed a penchant for antic humor, which kept him popular despite his silence. It also propelled him to the University of Iowa, the most famous center for stuttering research in the world. Around the country, speech pathology was fighting to be recognized as a science, and Iowa was the new discipline's polestar. Dozens of experiments were underway when Johnson arrived, and he enthusiastically threw himself into the invigorating work, switching to psychology for his masters study. "I became a speech pathologist because I needed one," he'd later say.

*Reprinted with permission of the New York Times, Inc., from *Times Magazine*, March 16, 2003.

Many of his fellow graduate students stuttered almost as painfully as he did, and they'd use one another as guinea pigs. They'd draw blood, hook themselves to electrodes, strike their knees to test reflexes, whip out notebooks in midstride and transcribe their own and others faltering speech. They'd administer electroshock and shoot guns off near each other's ears to see if being startled affected stuttering. (It didn't, although the same experiment performed on normal speakers did affect their speech.) They'd also put casts on one another's arms, since it was hoped that immobilizing a person's dominant hand somehow would untangle confused brain signals. At one point, about 30 students who stuttered, including Johnson, wandered the Iowa campus with their arms wrapped in plaster, sometimes playing badminton. "We knew that we were working on something central in the life of a human being," one of Johnson's contemporaries told an Iowa historian. "We weren't just puttering around on the fringes."

At the time, physiology had become the favored explanation at Iowa for stuttering. The department's lead professors were certain that the disorder originated in misdirected brain signals. They had used a new device called an electromyograph to study neuromuscular activity in people who stuttered, did not stutter and, in one experiment, people who were drunk (students who, solely in the interests of science, had become soused; the researchers skirted Prohibition by requisitioning alcohol from the university hospital.) The readouts from the booze-tinged subjects showed, to no one's surprise, impairment. Intriguingly, more comprehensive experiments showed that individuals who stuttered had subtle neuromuscular responses different from those of their fluent peers.

But Johnson, by 1937 an ambitious assistant professor, wasn't convinced. His life story suggested otherwise. He'd spoken fine until he was 5 or 6, when a teacher mentioned to his parents that he was starting to stutter. Gradually an obsession with his speech took hold. His voice grew hesitant. He self-consciously repeated sounds. Those, of course, are among the hallmarks of stammering. By worrying about the problem, he decided, he'd produced it. His disorder lay not in his brain, in biology, but in his learned behavior. Stuttering, he later concluded, "begins not in the child's mouth but in the parent's ear."

This idea was provocative and powerful, with enormous implications for speech therapy. If stuttering is learned behavior, it can be unlearned. Biography, however, isn't proof. Johnson, to validate his thesis, needed to design an experiment that induced stuttering. If, he reasoned, any and every child could he made to stutter, then obviously no underlying physiological defect was required. If stuttering could be called forth in normal youngsters, it would be proved as a learned, conditioned response.

In the fall of 1938, Wendell Johnson recruited one of his clinical psychology graduate students, 22-year-old Mary Tudor, who was avid but timorous, to undertake exactly that experiment. She was to study whether telling fluent children that they stuttered would make it so. Could she talk children into a speech defect? The university had an ongoing research relationship with an orphanage in Davenport, Iowa, so Johnson suggested she base her study there. And thus, on January 17, 1939, Mary Tudor drove along the high, swooping bluffs overlooking the Mississippi River to the Soldiers and Sailors Orphans' Home. She toted notepads, chalkboards, a Smedley dynamometer (to measure hand strength) and a cumbersome Dictaphone.

The study she began that morning is now the subject of a multimillion-dollar lawsuit against the State of Iowa and the University of Iowa. Despite its 64-year-old provenance, it has occasioned a spate of recent articles in newspapers and speech-sciences journals and a full-day symposium at the Graduate Center of the City University of New York in December (2002). Something happened at the orphanage in Davenport that seems to have been unintended by Johnson and not measurable by his science. Only now, at a remove of decades, can we begin to digest and appreciate what the Tudor study tells us about the origins of speech defects, as well as the ethics of science, the brittleness of children and the egos of driven men.

The Iowa Soldiers and Sailors Orphans' Home was founded as a refuge for the offspring of men killed in the Civil War. By 1939, at the height of the Great Depression, it housed more than 600 orphans and demi-orphans (those whose destitute parents, although alive, couldn't care for them) in clusters of small cottages. Not as harsh as the nearby Industrial School for Boys in Eldora, Iowa, or as forlorn as the Institute for Feeble-Minded Children at Glenwood, it was nevertheless spare, joyless and regimented. Children rose at 5:30 AM, had breakfast and cleaned until school began. They marched in long, careful lines, to facilitate order.

Mary Tudor's research at the Iowa Home began with the selection of 22 subjects. None were told the intent of her research. They believed that they were to receive speech therapy. Her experimental design was complicated. She was not only trying to induce stammering in healthy children; she was also trying to see whether telling individuals who stutter that their speech was fine would produce a change. Included among the 22 subjects were 10 orphans whom teachers and matrons had marked as stuttering before the study began. Tudor and five other graduate students who agreed to serve as judges listened to each of the children speak, graded them on a scale from 1 (poor) to 5 (fluent) and concurred with the school's assessment. "Unwilling to talk but certain definite 'stuttering' phenomena," a researcher wrote of one boy, "tension, prolongations, explosiveness, repetitions. A stutterer." The identified (ID) stuttering children were divided into two groups. Five were assigned to Group IA, the experimental set. They would be told:

"You do not stutter. Your speech is fine." The five in Group IB would serve as controls and be told, "Yes, your speech is as bad as people say."

The remaining 12 children were chosen at random from the population of normally fluent orphans. Six of these were assigned to Group IIA, the group that eventually would lead to the lawsuit and contention. These children, ranging in age from 5 to 15, were to be told that their speech was not normal at all, that they were beginning to stutter and that they must correct this immediately. The final six children in Group IIB, similar in age to those in Group I were normal speakers who were to be treated as such and given compliments on their nice enunciation.

On that first January visit, Tudor tested each child's I.Q. and handedness. A voguish theory then held that stuttering was caused by a cerebral imbalance. If, for example, you were born left-handed but were using your right hand, your nerve impulses would misfire, affecting your speech. Johnson felt the notion was nonsense, but he was thorough and suggested Tudor discern each child's handedness. She had them draw on chalkboard and squeeze the bulb of the dynamometer. Most were right-handed, but a sprinkling of lefties ran through all the groups. There was no correlation between handedness and speech in this subject crop. That was an auspicious start.

The experimental period lasted from January until late May 1939, and the actual intervention consisted of Tudor driving to Davenport from Iowa City every few weeks and talking with each child for about 45 minutes. She followed an agreed-upon script. In her dissertation, she reported that she talked to the stuttering youngsters who were going to be told that they did not stutter. She said to them, in part, "You'll outgrow [stuttering], and you will be able to speak even much better than you are speaking now . . . . Pay no attention to what others say about your speaking ability for undoubtedly they do not realize that this is only a phase."

To the fluent youngsters in (Group) IIA, who were to be branded as individuals who stutter, she said: "The staff has come to the conclusion that you have a great deal of trouble with your speech. . . . You have many of the symptoms of a child who is beginning to stutter. You must try to stop yourself immediately. Use your will power. . . . Do anything to keep from stuttering. . . . Don't ever speak unless you can do it right. You see how [name of a child in the institution who stuttered severely] stutters, don't you? Well, he undoubtedly started this very same way."

From the first, the children in (Group) IIA responded. After her second session with 5-year-old Norma Jean Pugh, Tudor wrote, "It was very difficult to get her to speak, although she spoke very freely the month before." Another in the group, 9-year-old Betty Romp, "practically refuses to talk," a researcher wrote in his final evaluation. "Held hand or arm over eyes most of the time." Hazel Potter, 15, the oldest in her group, became "much more conscious of herself, and she talked less," Tudor noted. Potter also began to interject and to snap her fingers in frustration. She was asked why she said /a/ so much. "Because I'm afraid I can't say the next word." Why did you snap your fingers? "Because I was afraid I was going to say /a/."

All of the children's schoolwork fell off. One of the boys began refusing to recite in class. The other, 11-year-old Clarence Fifer, a chubby, diffident child, started anxiously correcting himself. "He stopped and told me he was going to have trouble on words before he said them," Tudor reported. She asked him how he knew. He said that the sound "wouldn't come out. Feels like it's stuck in there."

The sixth orphan, Mary Korlaske, a 12-year-old, grew withdrawn and fractious. During their sessions, Tudor asked whether her best friend knew about her "stuttering." Korlaske muttered, "No." Why not? Korlaske shuffled her feet. "I hardly ever talk to her." Two years later, she ran away from the orphanage and eventually ended up at the rougher Industrial School for Girls. "I couldn't never tell my husband about it," Korlaske, now Mary Nixon, said in a brief telephone conversation in January. "It just ruined my life." Her voice broke. "I can't talk no more," she said, and with an audible oath, she hung up.

Mary Tudor herself wasn't untouched. Three times after her experiment had officially ended she returned to the orphanage to voluntarily provide follow-up care. She told the IIA children that they didn't stutter after all. The impact, however well-meaning, was questionable. She wrote to Johnson about the orphans in a slightly defensive letter dated April 22, 1940, "I believe that in time they . . . will recover, but we certainly made a definite impression on them." The emphasis is hers.

When Wendell Johnson was a boy, he ran the rounds of contemporary stuttering therapies. His family doctor gave him sugar pills. A faith healer, thundering from a high stage, frightened and disappointed him. He went to a chiropractor. At 16, with his speech almost unintelligible, he begged to be allowed to attend a far-off stuttering "school." There, for three months, he recited aloud in a deliberately flat monotone and swung dumbbells while metronomically chanting, "Have more backbone and less wishbone." None of this cured him, and abruptly, he quit. "I went to the station, stuttered to the ticket agent and to the conductor and . . . closed my eyes in despair," he wrote in *Because I Stutter*, his first book. "I was terribly ashamed . . . I hated stuttering."

His affliction shaped and spurred the remainder of his life and career. "Like most people who stutter, he was baffled by his stuttering," wrote Oliver Bloodstein, Ph.D., a professor emeritus of speech at Brooklyn College and Johnson's most distinguished pupil. "He spent hours trying to figure out what he was doing that made him stutter."

This lacerating curiosity drove him to undertake a series of ingenious experiments, before and after the Tudor study, into the essential nature of stammering itself. What is it? How does it work? To answer these questions, he began by giving individuals who stutter a page bordered in red and having them read aloud in front of an audience, where their stuttering would become worse. Afterward, the subjects tended to stutter painfully anytime they read a page marked with red, even when reading to a single person. Next, he blacked out words over which a particular stuttering reader had stumbled. When the person reached the word next to the one crossed out, he'd stutter. He'd become accustomed to stumbling there and, even without the troublesome word, he still did. These results said to Johnson that stuttering was indisputably a conditioned, learned response.

He also proved that individuals who stutter were consistent. They tended to stumble over the same sounds (although the sounds themselves varied from person to person) and grew to dread them, often substituting entire words. ("My f-f-fa . . . dad.") They'd also whisper. When they were about to reach troublesome fricatives, their eyes would bulge. They'd thump their knees, click their fingers, rasp desperately or shake their heads in a spasmodic attempt to force out the sound. Johnson defined those actions as the associated behaviors of stuttering and claimed that in adults they would diminish if the individual who stuttered relaxed and didn't anticipate a speech block. He liked to point out that in certain situations even the most afflicted don't stutter, during, for instance, singing or in unpressured speech with infants or dogs. "One person who stuttered severely virtually lived the life of a nomad because he was able to communicate vocally only whenever he established himself in a new town," wrote Oliver Bloodstein, who did Johnson's fieldwork.

Johnson's findings about the nature of stuttering, once it has begun, remain the accepted wisdom to this day. The disorder does respond to conditioning, and once established, stuttering can have a ruinous momentum. Often, the worse someone stutters, the more he fears speaking, and the worse his speech becomes.

What Johnson's thinking did not explain is why severe stuttering starts. Episodes of speech disfluency are common among adults and children, especially the very young. But about 5 percent of all youngsters exhibit clinical stammering, according to Ehud Yairi, a professor of speech and hearing science at the

University of Illinois. Of these, about 75 percent recover without treatment, but about 1 percent of all people (about three million Americans) continue to stutter noticeably into adulthood. It is those whom Johnson studied in his work on the progression of the disorder. Why, though, were those few stricken in the first place?

Johnson had no family history of stuttering and dismissed the possibility that the condition could be heritable. "Stuttering is learned behavior, Johnson said, and he repeated it again and again," Bloodstein wrote in an E-mail message. "It virtually became his mantra." He had indirect, anecdotal data, too, that backed his contention. Beginning in 1934, he and his assistants questioned the mothers of dozens of youngsters who stuttered, asking when the disorder had begun and how the family had responded. He also tested age-matched fluent speakers and found that they had many speech defects as well. Unfortunately for the "stutterers," Johnson said, their parents overreacted, made the children panic and produced full-blown stuttering. The diagnosis caused the condition. Johnson termed this the diagnosogenic theory, and it became the cornerstone for his writing and teaching, his growing fame and eventually the basis for his ideas about the treatment of stuttering children. It also, by its dictates, should have ensured that all the orphans in Mary Tudor's Group IIA would stutter soon after Tudor began telling them that they did.

But they did not. In fact, the most telling aspect of Mary Tudor's experiment is that it failed completely. Of the six normal children who were falsely labeled as individuals who stutter, two actually improved their speech fluency, according to the researchers' ratings, over the course of the five-month study—one by almost a full point, from 3 to 3.8. Another's fluency rose from 3 to 3.6. For two others, their fluency ratings didn't budge. Of the two children whose fluency fell, one, Clarence Fifer, dropped from 2.6 to 2, the second, Hazel Potter, from 3.1 to 2.8.

The other primary study group fared little better. Of the children who actually stuttered who were told they now spoke fine, two showed slight improvements in fluency, two decreased in fluency and one was unchanged. The results for each of the groups were "not only insignificant, but also in the wrong (unexpected) direction," concluded Yairi and a colleague in an article in the May 2002 issue of *The American Journal of Speech-Language Pathology*.

The experiment did, however, have an impact. In each case, the fluent children of Group IIA began to act like individuals who stutter. "All of the children in this group showed overt behavioral changes," Mary Tudor wrote in her thesis, "that were in the direction of the types of inhibitive, sensitive, embarrassed reactions shown by many adult stutterers in reaction to their speech. There was a tendency for them to become less talkative." They also, during their sessions with her and in front of the researchers, shuffled their feet, whispered, snapped their fingers, gulped, gasped and clamped their mouths shut. They looked like people who stutter. They spoke fine.

It seems highly unlikely that you can make a person stutter. You can induce the accompanying tics—the shuffling and the self-consciousness. Those can be taught and reinforced. But clinical stuttering cannot. It exists or it doesn't. Johnson's theory was not upheld.

After Mary Tudor submitted her completed masters thesis in August 1939 with a dedication to Johnson, it sank straightaway into obscurity. Johnson did not oversee its publication, as he often did with his students' theses. He did not include it in his otherwise comprehensive indexes of University of Iowa stuttering research. Not until 2001 did it receive national press attention, in a series of articles in *The San Jose Mercury News*. However, the thesis, which was available at the university library, did have a ghost life among Iowa speech pathology students. "Those who had heard about it nicknamed it the Monster Study," remembers Franklin Silverman, a professor of speech pathology at Marquette University and a former student of Johnson's. "It reminded people of the Nazi experiments on human subjects. The other professors at the time told him that it would ruin his reputation to publish the data. It was chilling and disturbing, especially to think that Wendell Johnson, of all people, had sanctioned it. He knew the pain of being told that you stutter."

It is an ugly thing, after all, to experiment on orphans. And Johnson's admirers, who still are legion, struggle to understand why he proposed and designed the project. "I have to assume it was because he firmly believed that it would serve a greater good, that it would help thousands of other children who stuttered and that any damage would be temporary and reversible," says D. C. Spriestersbach, Vice President and Dean Emeritus of the University of Iowa and another of Johnson's students. "He was a wonderful, empathetic man, and he understood the torment of a speech defect. He wouldn't have been able to bear it if he thought he'd actually forced someone to stutter."

He pauses. "But he never talked about the Tudor study to me or anyone else that I'm aware of. So all I can do really is guess."

During the 1940s, when Johnson, despite his speech impairment, was one of the most popular lecturers on the Iowa campus, he used to exhort his students to question "the voice of authority." He'd say, "Whenever you hear a dogmatic, absolutist statement from any kind of 'expert,' ask, 'What do you mean and how do you know?'"

The Tudor study was not only morally troubling; its results must have been, for Johnson, confounding. The data threatened to undercut his belief, which was unswerving, that stuttering is purely behavioral. "It ran counter to what he stood for," says Gerald Zimmermann, a former speech professor at Iowa and now a literacy specialist. "I wouldn't want to publicize a blow like that either. But, hey, that's science."

Johnson sometimes referred to the study in lectures, claiming that it had caused an orphan, presumably Hazel Potter, to stutter and therefore validated his diagnosogenic ideas. But the researchers, in their final evaluation, graded her as someone who did not stutter.

Johnson did not mention the study again. In 1959, he published his famous *The Onset of Stuttering*, which laid out the diagnosogenic theory in detail. However, nowhere in its pages does he mention the orphan experiment. The Tudor study "should have been discussed," Zimmermann says. "It should have been part of the record and the canon. Maybe everyone would have supported the diagnosogenic theory anyway. Johnson was persuasive. But at least a question would have been raised."

From the 1950s until the early 1980s, Johnson's theory, unsullied by doubts, was the underpinning of most childhood speech intervention in America. Therapists, swayed by diagnosogenic theory, declined to work directly with youngsters who stuttered, fearing that the therapy could worsen the affliction. They'd instead counsel a child's parents, telling them to stop worrying so much. Sometimes this helped the child. Other times it didn't.

Today, one of the most widely accepted models for explaining persistent stuttering is that a genetic component provides a biological predisposition to stutter. Not everyone with "stuttering genes" progresses, of course, to a full-blown disorder. There are environmental cues that are necessary. One of these may be a panic-stricken parent. In a child with a sensitive temperament, a father or mother's reaction may push the child over the edge. In this way, Wendell Johnson's thesis partly survives. But as the sole predictor of stuttering, diagnosogenic theory has been thoroughly overthrown. "No one believes anymore that only your parents make you stutter," says Robert Goldfarb, head of the Ph.D. program in speech and hearing sciences at the CUNY Graduate Center and the organizer of the symposium there. "It's probably a shame for speech therapy and for parents that anyone ever did."

Nowadays, researchers think that the most helpful form of speech therapy is working directly with children. In face-to-face sessions with their therapists, children are encouraged to practice breath control, easing words out instead of forcing them and stretch out sounds to make them longer. One can't help wondering what would have happened had Johnson published the Tudor findings. Would the results have raised issues that might have led to an earlier shift in treatment for stuttering children? And would those youngsters who stuttered have been better served by this more direct intervention? We can't know. Though researchers now have more success reducing disfluency in children, the discipline of speech therapy remains inexact and, for some who stutter, eternally ineffective. "We don't have any way of measuring the impact of having lost the Tudor study for all those years," Zimmermann says.

Perhaps Johnson felt the need to protect a doctrine that explained not only a crippling affliction but also the very arc of his life. Wendell Johnson "was outgoing," Oliver Bloodstein wrote. "He was comradely. But he was also hard at work for recognition in his field . . . like so many gifted people, he was burdened with an unshakable conviction that he was right."

The reverberations of the 64-year-old Tudor study will sound for years. The three surviving orphans from Group IIA, Norma Jean Pugh (now Kathryn Meacham), Mary Korlaske (now Mary Nixon) and Hazel Potter (now Hazel Dornbush), are each suing the State and University of Iowa for millions of dollars, citing among other things the infliction of emotional distress and fraudulent misrepresentation. The estates of the three deceased orphans will be part of the suit. "I think that a jury will agree that even if these people's speech wasn't exactly ruined, their lives were," says Evan Douthit, a Kansas City, Missouri attorney who is representing five of the claimants. "Kathryn Meacham has thought of herself as a freak all her life. She still hates to talk, except to her family and a few people in her church. She's a sad, sad lady."

Hazel Potter Dornbush is scrappy and decisive at 79. "Imagine trying to wreck a little child's voice," she says. "But I've moved on. I married a good man. I talk O.K. Even the orphanage wasn't that bad. There were always other children around, so it wasn't lonely." She pauses. "I don't really remember being that close to any," she adds, suddenly puzzled. "But back then, you know, I was quiet."

In 1965, at 59, Wendell Johnson sat at his desk still defending diagnosogenic theory. He was preparing an entry for the *Encyclopaedia Britannica* on "Speech Disorders" when he suffered a massive heart attack. The 4,000-word essay, completed and published posthumously, brooks no dissent. "The child learns speech-disruptive behavior as he tries to keep from stuttering and so to gain approval," he writes. Johnson's didacticism lessens near the end, however, and he grows almost gentle. "Persons with speech disorders . . . have traditionally known the scorn, ridicule and even revulsion of their society," he writes in the voice of a man driven all his life to make sense of the ability to speak.

2

DIAGNOSIS

Robert Goldfarb, Ph.D.

One of the most thoroughly studied, and most frequently misunderstood, of all the disorders of speech and language is stuttering. The hypothesis that stuttering is basically an organic disorder is at least as old as Aristotle, who considered the problem to relate to the structure of the individual's tongue (Goldfarb, 1985). Theories about both the onset of stuttering and the moment of stuttering have abounded, ranging from inherited predisposition to psychoanalytic theories to cybernetic models. The definitive analysis of stuttering has not yet been written, and it may be that stuttering will ultimately be found to represent a group of symptoms and behaviors, and no single description or treatment will be sufficient.

Stuttering Versus Normal Disfluency in Young Children

Diagnosis and treatment of stuttering, at least from the 1920s through the 1970s in the United States, tended to follow protocols developed at the University of Iowa. Parent counseling was seen as both necessary and sufficient treatment for stuttering in young children. This view was likely an outgrowth of Wendell Johnson's *semantogenic/diagnosogenic theory*, which held that the kind of speech shown by children who stutter at the onset of stuttering is not distinguishable from normal disfluency. Johnson (1955) noted that the stuttering label tended to be applied to a child, who may have been normally disfluent, by nonprofessionals such as parents. When parents themselves stuttered, Johnson suggested they were overly sensitive to disfluencies heard in their child's speech, thus offering one explanation of why stuttering tends to run in families. Parental attitudes "fostered the child's belief that speaking is a difficult task, requiring mental and physical effort, and that it must be produced precisely, quickly, and maturely" (Conture, 1982, p. 163). Around the same time as Johnson's publication (Glasner & Rosenthal, 1957), the diagnosogenic theory was depicted as an oversimplification. The parent's role was seen as a source of supplementary environmental stress, rather than the cause of the disfluency.

Johnson (1955, 1959) grouped repetitions of phrases and whole words together with syllabic repetitions to form the conclusion that the parents of children who stutter and the parents of children who do not reported the same kinds of disfluency in their children's speech. Subsequent research has shown that syllabic repetitions tend to distinguish the disfluent behaviors of children who do and do not stutter (Van Riper, 1982). In addition, Van Riper's (1982) "A to Z" list of behaviors associated with stuttering included the presence of more than two syllable repetitions per one hundred words (fewer than two syllable repetitions in normal disfluency); and the presence of prolongations that last longer than one second in stuttering (and less than one second in normal disfluency).

Bloodstein (1960) proposed a *continuity hypothesis* in which behaviors commonly described as stuttering cannot distinguish stuttering as a problem from disfluencies in normal speaking children, who also may show these behaviors. Most young children will stutter sometime. Those who were eventually labeled as stuttering were those who stuttered severely and persistently. Therefore, diagnosis, according to the continuity hypothesis, is a futile and meaningless exercise. In contrast, Johannsen, Schulze, and Wallesch (1989) considered differential diagnosis between stuttering and normal disfluency to be essential, because the disorder is more difficult to treat in adolescents and adults.

Characteristics of Stuttering

Before attempting to assess the presence or absence of stuttering in young children, it is important to establish an operational definition of stuttering. The World Health Organization (1977) definition of stuttering was used by Andrews et al. (1983) in their exhaustive review of research findings and theories. Accordingly, stuttering is considered to be a disorder in the rhythm of speech in which the individual knows precisely what he or she wishes to say but, at the time, is unable to say it because of an involuntary, repetitive prolongation or cessation of a sound. These are also called *disfluencies*, which are disruptions or breaks in the smooth flow of speech (Ambrose & Yairi, 1999). Johnson's (1959) categorization of eight different disfluency types—interjections, revisions, incomplete phrases, phrase repetitions, word repetitions, part-word repetitions, prolonged sounds, and broken words—was incorporated as part of a procedure for the automatic recognition of disfluencies in the speech of children who stutter (Glenn, Howell, & Sackin, 1997). In describing young children who stutter, Conture (1982) focused on within-word speech disfluencies. These included sound/syllable repetitions, sound prolongations, and within-word pauses.

Perkins, Kent, and Curlee (1991) offered a definition of stuttering which may permit verification in the speech science laboratory. They referred to stuttering as a speech disruption where the speaker has lost control of the ability to initiate or continue an utterance. The resulting acoustic events provide a standard on which to base perceptual definitions of stuttering. The speech science laboratory has not yet been effective in prognostic assessment of stuttering. In examining 58 children who stutter, Brosch, Häge, and Johannsen (2001) were unable to relate acoustic analysis with clinical measurements of stuttering.

Nonspeech characteristics (see "associated symptoms" below) may be observed in many individuals who stutter. Extraneous body movements are displayed in association with, and often at the same time as, disfluencies. Bloodstein (1995) noted that the orofacial mechanism is prominently involved, and may include blinking the eyes, wrinkling the forehead, frowning, quivering the nostrils, distorting the mouth, exhaling suddenly, and/or jerking the head. Less frequently involved are movements of the hands, arms, legs, and/or torso.

Normal Disfluency in Preschool Children

Most young speakers exhibit disfluencies occasionally, and even characteristically. Preschoolers tend to repeat sounds, syllables, words, and phrases and may also interject syllables, words, and phrases. They may revise a thought, pause at places other than phrase boundaries, prolong sounds, and produce incomplete phrases. The development of syntactic skills may also adversely affect fluency, as children are most disfluent at the beginning of syntactic units, and when the length and complexity of their utterances increase. Pragmatic factors, such as pressures of competition and excitement when speaking may also increase disfluency (Guitar, 1998).

Differential Diagnosis

The discovery of disfluencies is necessary, but not sufficient, to differentiate normal from pathologic conditions. In fact, the presence of disfluencies in young children is not considered abnormal, unusual, or even uncommon. There is a basic question of quantitative differences or qualitative differences in arriving at a diagnosis of stuttering; in fact, both are important, even at the earliest stages of stuttering. There is essential agreement in the literature regarding general principles for differential diagnosis, although the specifics often differ.

One fruitful procedure (Yaruss, LaSalle, & Conture, 1998) involved a three-part evaluation: conversational interaction between child and caregiver(s) (20 to 30 minutes); evaluation of the child's speech, language, and related behaviors (60 to 90 minutes); and an interview of the child's caregiver(s) (45 to 60 minutes). This three-hour procedure may be unrealistic in many work settings. However, the traditional method of assessing a wide variety of interacting psychosocial, psycholinguistic, and physiologic variables will likely take longer and may not differentiate among children at risk for stuttering.

Yaruss et al. (1998) used measures of speech fluency, measures of speech and language development, and other measures, including the child's diadochokinetic rate and parents' speaking rates to determine presence of a pathologic condition. "Not surprisingly" (Yaruss et al., 1998, p. 72), children referred for treatment had a significantly higher frequency of disfluency, a tendency toward sound prolongations rather than repetitions, and higher stuttering severity scores. The authors hastened to note that there was still considerable overlap between children recommended for re-evaluation and those who received neither treatment nor re-evaluation. "It would seem essentially impossible to develop absolute criteria for determining which children should receive which diagnostic recommendation" (Yaruss et al., 1998, p. 72).

The Initial Evaluation

Whether or not normal disfluency may be absolutely distinguished from incipient or actual stuttering, it is important to obtain baseline measures. Pre- and post-therapy assessments provide evidence of response to treatment. During the initial evaluation, the clinician should obtain written permission to audiotape and videotape the evaluation so that disfluencies and associated behaviors can be reviewed and analyzed. Bring a manual stopwatch as well. Measuring the duration of disfluencies is a diagnostic indicator of the presence of stuttering. For example, an average of the three longest stuttering blocks is used in scoring the *Stuttering Severity Instrument* (SSI-3; Riley, 1980). If more sophisticated instrumentation is available, more accurate measures of stuttering may be obtained. The Speech Spectrographic Display (SSD) was used in a study (Zebrowski, 1991) of duration of speech disfluencies. Acoustic measurement of duration is not affected by human reaction time, compared to duration measurements with a manual stopwatch. The following are critical elements of the initial evaluation.

Case History

The purpose of a case history is to identify individuals and situations associated with the onset and the moment of stuttering. It usually involves family background, health and developmental history, detailed information regarding circumstances and time of onset of stuttering, and characteristics of the moment of stuttering (Yairi & Ambrose, 1992). It may also be useful to know the child's hearing and visual acuity, as well as contact information for the child's school and teacher. Written questionnaires, such as the one used in *The Stocker Probe for Fluency and Language* (Stocker & Goldfarb, 1995), may be mailed at the time the appointment is scheduled. The same information may also be obtained by interviewing the child's parents, family members, teachers, and/or caregivers. These individuals should also be encouraged to discuss their attitudes toward the child's disfluencies.

Speech Sample

Protocols for collection of speech samples may be found in Yaruss, LaSalle, and Conture (1998), noted above. Videotaping these sessions will facilitate subsequent analysis of data. In the parent-child interaction, the parent evokes natural conversation from the child using age-appropriate toys and books. The second interaction, between clinician and client, may include formal assessment instruments, such as the SSI-3 (Riley, 1980) and the Stocker Probe (Stocker & Goldfarb, 1995).

Analysis of the Speech Sample

The analysis includes quantitative and qualitative measures of speech disfluencies, including frequency, type, and duration of disfluencies. Rate of speech and severity of stuttering are terminal goals of analysis.

Disfluency Type

The clinician needs to understand what the child is doing to interfere with talking, how the child's disfluencies have changed over time, and how these changes might be related to the child's compensatory speech production strategies (Zebrowski, 2000). Differentiating normal disfluency from stuttering may be supported by noting the proportion of different disfluency types produced by the child. These types of disfluencies may be categorized as *within-word* disfluencies, which include monosyllabic whole-word repetitions, sound/syllable repetitions, audible sound prolongations, or inaudible sound prolongations and *between-word* disfluencies, which include polysyllabic whole-word repetitions, phrase repetitions, revisions, and interjections, based on guidelines provided by Yaruss et al. (1998), who recorded these disfluency types on a count sheet. Studies that compare the speech of young children who stutter and normally disfluent children (Yairi & Ambrose, 1992) reveal that children who stutter produce more within-word disfluencies, such as sound/syllable repetitions and sound prolongations, than children who do not stutter. The difference is more quantitative than qualitative, as all children tend to produce the same kinds of speech disfluencies. The same study indicated that children who produce a minimum of three within-word speech disfluencies in one hundred syllables of running conversational speech are at higher risk for developing stuttering.

Frequency of Disfluency

Initial baseline and baseline recovery measures of stuttering typically include overall frequency of disfluency as a basis of documenting broad improvement in therapy. A frequency count tends to ignore type of disfluency, and is determined by simply counting the number of disfluent words per total words in the speech sample. It may also be represented somewhat more accurately in fraction form, with "syllables stuttered" as the numerator and "syllables spoken" as the denominator. As a diagnostic measure it may provide some information about the extent to which the child disrupts the flow of speech.

Duration

Duration of sound prolongations as well as sound or syllable repetitions may indicate presence and severity of stuttering (Van

Riper, 1982). A sound prolongation lasting more than one second tends to indicate stuttering (and not normal disfluency) in preschool and school-age children. In scaling severity of stuttering (e.g., Riley, 1980), a one-second sound prolongation represents moderate stuttering. However, a sound prolongation of one-half second duration does not differentiate children whose onset of stuttering occurred within 12 months from those children who do not stutter (Zebrowski, 1991).

Severity

Particularly when applied to children who stutter, severity ratings are subjective. Attempts to use objective measures of stuttering in published assessment tools for young children (e.g., Riley, 1980; Stocker & Goldfarb, 1995) include frequency, type, and duration of stuttering, together with physical concomitants, as well as level of communicative demand. These measures fall short of a reasonable expectation of objectivity, because of the variability of stuttering in young children. Although we acknowledge the usefulness of documenting the above behaviors, current severity measures probably are not more helpful or prescriptive for intervention than a classical description, such as Bloodstein's (1960) four phases of stuttering, a progressive classification of severity, or Van Riper's (1982) four tracks, which stress developmental variability in stuttering.

Associated Symptoms

Physical manifestations concomitant to the vocal aspect of disfluency are usually termed "secondary behaviors." They are visible or audible physical behaviors that accompany repetitions and prolongations. Secondary behaviors should not be confused with the "secondary" stage of stuttering (first reported by Bluemel, 1932), where the child becomes aware of the social consequences of disfluency. To avoid confusion, use Bloodstein's (1995) description of "associated symptoms" to describe features that do not include repetitions, prolongations, or pauses. These concomitant features may appear amazing in their variety, and include "(1) visible or audible reactions accompanying or interspersed among stutterers' speech interruptions, (2) visceral or physiological correlates of stuttering, and (3) changes in stutter-ers' perceptions of their environment and in their subjective states when experiencing difficulty with speech" (Bloodstein, 1995, p. 19). A brief list of associated symptoms would include eye movement of varying types; head, torso, and limb move-ment; as well as noisy breathing, vocal pitch changes, whistling, jaw jerking, tongue protruding, lip pressing, and tension in the muscles of mastication, lips, and in the strap muscles of the neck.

Assessment of Stuttering in Older Children and Adults

The main objectives of an assessment of stuttering in older children and adults are similar to those for stuttering in young children. The clinician begins by obtaining history of the disorder and its development; learning and describing the overt behaviors asso-ciated with the moment of stuttering; determining which covert behaviors, such as negative emotional responses and mental con-structs, cause or maintain the overt behaviors; assessing associated motor behaviors; and recommending whether further interven-tion, such as follow-up evaluation or therapy, is warranted.

Core behaviors refer to the basic, involuntary, observable behaviors of stuttering, which include part- and whole-word repetitions, prolongations, and stoppages of air. Associated symptoms are typically described in such operant terms as avoidance and escape, where the individual attempts to deal with the aversive consequences of stuttering. Attempts to exit the stutter and finish the word may be accompanied by eye blinks, head nods, and interjection of sounds (escape responses). Pauses, word substitutions, and hand movements are attempts to prevent stuttering (avoidance responses). In mentalistic terms, these behaviors often result in internalized feelings of shame and embarrassment.

Implications of Diagnosis for Treatment

Through the early 1970s, a major focus of clinical management of stuttering, particularly in young children, consisted of counsel-ing parents/caregivers. There were lists of "do's" and "don'ts."

The former included treating with customary love and affection, encouraging speech during periods of fluency, and removing speech-related pressures. Caregivers were also admonished to avoid cutting off the individual's speech during a block, refraining from telling the individual to "slow down," and not referring to labored speech as "stuttering." From the 1980s to the present, a more direct approach took favor. Stuttering was seen to be especially alterable in its early stages. Spontaneous recovery was seen as an oversold notion. Direct modification of stuttered speech when it first appears was deemed important and effective, resulting in operant-based treatments. Finally, the use of breath stream management and prolonged speech effectively induced the individual who stutters to "slow down."

Conclusion

Traditionally, evaluation of an individual's stuttering etiology considered the interaction of physiologic, psychologic, psychosocial, psycholinguistic, and environmental factors. That is, stuttering could not be understood without examining the person who stutters, the social context within which the person communicates, and the interaction of environmentally generated communicative demands and the speaker's individual capacity for speech fluency. Although we do not deny the usefulness of reports that may be obtained from a licensed psychologist, we recommend an assessment model that does not require that we either refer to other professionals or step outside our scope of practice. Following is a model (Santo Pietro & Goldfarb, 1995, pp. 13–14), based on set theory, originally used in describing assessment and treatment of aphasia in adults. In mathematics, the intersection of two sets consists of the elements the sets have in common. Areas of assessing a person who stutters are grouped according to the intersections in the drawing, or Venn diagram, in Figure 2–1A.

The diagram portrays a person with a fluency impairment communicating with a communication partner within an environment. None of the component sets should be assessed independently of the others. Furthermore, the approach to assessment is best conceived in terms of the intersection it targets. For exam-

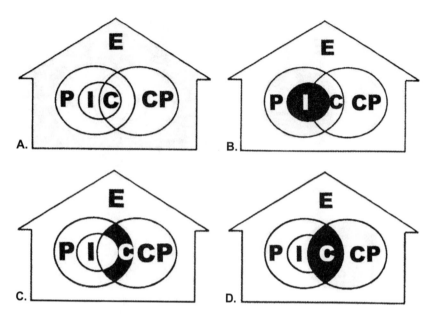

Figure 2–1. **A.** A model portraying a person (P) with a fluency impairment (I) communicating (C) with a communication partner (CP) within an environment (E). The intersection of sets contains the elements the sets have in common. Due to the overlapping nature of the elements within this model, each component in the model should not be assessed independently of the others. **B.** A model of therapy and assessment confined to circle I, impairment, which may be considered *treating to deficit*. **C.** A model of therapy that strives to maximize the person's unimpaired communication skills. **D.** A model of therapy that repairs communication acts between a person who stutters and the communication partner. *(continues)*

ple, if you focus on the vocal and motor characteristics of the individual's stuttering, you are working on impairment [I]. However, [I] is contained completely within the set of the person [P], who is contained completely within an environment [E]. It also intersects the communication [C] between the person who stutters and the communication partner [CP], as well as the communication partner as an individual, as seen in Figure 2–1B.

Assessing and treating stuttering will have a direct effect on the total person [P], the communication partner [CP], the level of communication between them [C], and their shared

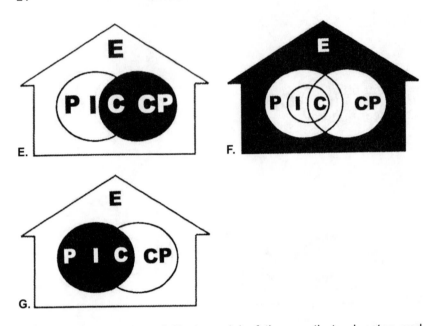

Figure 2–1. *(continued)* **E.** A model of therapy that educates and supports communication partners. **F.** A model of therapy that repairs the communication-impaired environment and provides opportunities for communication. **G.** A model of therapy that treats the whole person to reduce psychosocial handicap. (From *Techniques for aphasia rehabilitation generating effective treatment* [p. 13–14], by M.J. Santo Pietro & R. Goldfarb,1995, Vero Beach, FL: The Speech Bin. Copyright 1995 by The Speech Bin. Adapted with permission.)

environment [E]. Conversely, [P], [CP], [C], and [E] will have a direct effect on the level of impairment as therapy proceeds. Therapy and assessment must not be confined to circle [I], which may be considered *treating to deficit*. To be effective, treatment should address all the other intersections in the diagram to maximize the person's unimpaired communication skills (*treating to strength*) (Figure 2–1C), repair communication acts between children who stutter and their communication partners (Figure 2–1D), educate and support communication partners (Figure 2–1E), repair the communication-impaired environment and provide opportunities for communication (Figure 2–1F), and treat the whole person to reduce psychosocial handicap (Figure 2–1G).

There are two major points of applying set theory:

1. Diagnosis of stuttering must be comprehensive. The whole person as well as the communication partners and environment must be treated.

2. The individual's needs and wishes must be an integral component in determining approaches to treatment.

The Received Wisdom Versus The Awful Truth: A Pseudo-Bayesian Conclusion

The received wisdom claimed vociferous support for a variety of organismic, or environmental, or interactional models to provide a theoretical basis for the onset, or the cause of, stuttering. The awful truth is that, perhaps unique among communication disorders, the study of stuttering currently proceeds from an atheoretical basis (see Chapter 8 of this book). Frequent references to the work of Bloodstein support a consideration of him as the world's foremost living authority on stuttering. At the same time, though, by virtue of including a section on diagnosing stuttering in children, this book is required to reject his continuity hypothesis.

References

Ambrose, N., & Yairi, E. (1999). Normative disfluency data for early childhood stuttering. *Journal of Speech, Language, and Hearing Research, 42,* 895–909.

Andrews, G., Crain, A., Feyer, A., Hoddinot, B., Howie, P., & Neilson, M. (1983). Stuttering: A review of research findings and theories circa 1982. *Journal of Speech and Hearing Disorders, 48,* 226–246.

Bloodstein, O. (1960). The development of stuttering. II. Developmental phases. *Journal of Speech and Hearing Disorders, 25,* 366–376.

Bloodstein, O. (1995). *A handbook on stuttering* (5th ed.). San Diego: Singular Publishing Group.

Bluemel, C. S. (1932). Primary and secondary stammering. *Quarterly Journal of Speech, 18,* 187–200.

Brosch, S., Häge, A., & Johannson, H. (2001). Value of acoustic speech analysis for prognostic assessment of stuttering in children. Partial results of a prospective longitudinal study. *HNO, 49,* 289–297.

Conture, E. G. (1982). Youngsters who stutter: Diagnosis, parent counseling and referral. *Journal of Developmental and Behavioral Pediatrics, 3*, 163–169.

Glasner, P. J., & Rosenthal, D. (1957). Parental diagnosis of stuttering in young children. *Journal of Speech and Hearing Disorders, 22*, 288–295.

Glenn, K., Howell, P., & Sakin, S. (1997). Development of a two-stage procedure for the automatic recognition of disfluencies in the speech of children who stutter: Psychometric procedures appropriate for selection of training material for lexical disfluency classifiers. *Journal of Speech, Language, and Hearing Research, 40*, 1073–1084.

Goldfarb, R. (1985). Speech handicaps/communication disorders. In T. Husen & T. N. Postlethwaite (Eds.), *International encyclopedia of education* (pp. 4760–4766). Oxford: Pergamon.

Guitar, B. (1998). *Stuttering: An integrated approach to its nature and treatment* (2nd ed.). Baltimore: Williams & Wilkins.

Johannsen, H., Schulze, H., & Wallesch, B. (1989). Stuttering in children as a problem of phoniatric outpatient clinics. *Auris, Nasus, Larynx, 16*(Suppl. 1), S91–S109.

Johnson, W. (1955). *Stuttering in children and adults.* Minneapolis: University of Minnesota Press.

Johnson, W. (1959). *The onset of stuttering.* Minneapolis: University of Minnesota Press.

Perkins, W. H., Kent, R. D., & Curlee, R .F. (1991). A theory of neuropsycholinguistic function in stuttering. *Journal of Speech and Hearing Research, 34*, 734–752.

Riley, G. D. (1980). *Stuttering severity instrument for children and adults.* Austin, TX: Pro-Ed.

Santo Pietro, M. J., & Goldfarb, R. (1995). *Techniques for aphasia rehabilitation generating effective treatment.* Vero Beach, FL: The Speech Bin.

Stocker, B., & Goldfarb, R. (1995). *The Stocker probe for fluency and language* (3rd ed.). Vero Beach, FL: The Speech Bin.

Yairi, E., & Ambrose, N. (1992). Onset of stuttering in preschool children: Selected factors. *Journal of Speech and Hearing Research, 35*, 782–788.

Yaruss, J. S., LaSalle, L. R., & Conture, E. G. (1998). Evaluating stuttering in young children: Diagnostic data. *American Journal of Speech-Language Pathology, 7*, 62–76.

Van Riper, C. (1982). *The nature of stuttering* (2nd ed.). Englewood Cliffs, NJ: Prentice-Hall.

Zebrowski, P. (1991). Duration of the speech disfluencies of beginning stutterers. *Journal of Speech and Hearing Research, 34*, 483–491.

Zebrowski, P. (2000). Stuttering. In J. B. Tomblin, H. L. Morris, & D. C. Spriestersbach (Eds.), *Diagnosis in speech-language pathology* (2nd ed., pp. 199–231). San Diego: Singular Publishing Group.

3

RESEARCH IN STUTTERING AT THE UNIVERSITY OF IOWA CIRCA 1939

Oliver Bloodstein, Ph.D.

Johnson may be best known as the author of the diagnosogenic theory, but he was much more than that. He was the foremost researcher on stuttering of his day, and much of what we know about stuttering is due to studies that he directed. Meaningful research comes from compelling ideas, and Johnson was above all a pursuer of ideas. It was an idea that led him to the Tudor study, the notion that evaluative labeling can influence behavior. There is some question about whether the diagnosogenic theory was then fully formed in his mind; but when I came to Iowa a few years later, he was citing Tudor's study in his lectures in support of the theory. To the best of my recollection, he told us that one child actually did begin to stutter as a result of the procedure. However, the child was said to have stopped stuttering after some speech therapy, and for most of us that was enough to allay any discomfort we might have felt about the study. At least I do not remember being shocked or hearing expressions of dismay from any of the other students. Besides, we would have forgiven Johnson for almost anything. Nevertheless, Johnson must have had some qualms about the ethics of the study. He never published it.

What made him do it? Johnson, in his thirties, was a much liked and admired teacher. He was outgoing. He was comradely. His students called him Jack. But he was also hard at work for recognition in his field. He had an unusual new theory of stuttering and, like so many gifted people, he was burdened with an unshakable conviction that he was right. I once looked up stuttering in the 1968 edition of the *Encyclopaedia Britannica*. There I found an article by Johnson that was essentially an exposition of the diagnosogenic theory with almost no hint that there was any difference of opinion about stuttering in the field. And when I wrote something that deviated somewhat from the diagnosogenic view, he told some of his students, "Oliver has been away from Iowa too long." Perhaps this helps to some extent to explain why Johnson did the Tudor study. A man who was so firmly convinced that he was right could easily have convinced himself that the study would do no harm.

The Tudor study certainly does not offer proof of the diagnosogenic theory. Johnson attempted to find that proof in three investigations that he directed over a period of years. The theory is technically very difficult to verify directly. To do so, researchers would have to be stationed close by at the moment children are first diagnosed as stuttering by their parents in order to determine whether their disfluency is or is not perfectly normal. The method Johnson chose was to study the speech of young stuttering and normal speaking children and to interview their parents. This yielded a large amount of data on children's disfluencies and home backgrounds. In 1959, Johnson collected all of this information in a book entitled *The Onset of Stuttering*. As expected, the data showed that the children who stuttered were more disfluent than the children who did not stutter. Aside from that, the most prominent conclusion that the data supported was that there was not a single type or feature of disfluency that was not shared by at least some of the children in both groups. This even extended to signs of effort and emotional reactions. Johnson summed this up by stating that there is no natural line of demarcation between the disfluencies of young children who do and do not stutter. In my view, this is a very important conclusion, but it is not easily reconciled with Johnson's theory. The theory says that stuttering begins as the effort to avoid normal disfluency. There is no continuity between a thing and the avoidance of the thing; they are clearly demarcated from each other. Johnson was finally led to state that incipient stuttering was not a feature of a child's speech, but a "problem" that arises for a listener. Which led Robert West to remark that my old teacher "certainly draws his ideas out to gossamer thinness."

In short, the Iowa studies did not produce convincing evidence for the diagnosogenic theory. But that research was not Johnson's major contribution. His enduring contribution as a researcher had to do with the origin of a stuttering block, which is something quite different. When we ask what causes stuttering, we are usually referring to the conditions under which the disorder begins. But the question has another meaning. Here is a young man who has been stuttering for 20 years. If he is like most people who stutter, he does not stutter all the time. In fact he is likely to say most of his words normally. But now he has a block. Why? There must be a reason. What is happening? Or as Johnson preferred to put it, "What is he doing?" What is the nature of this thing we call a stuttering block? In an effort to answer this question Johnson embarked on a program of research on the factors that govern the occurrence of stutterings. In the course of this research, he and his students discovered almost all the basic facts we know about the subject.

Characteristically, he was motivated in this research by an idea. It was the concept that stuttering blocks arise from belief in the imagined difficulty of speech. This was an idea that had been broached long before in different forms. Johnson found it compatible with his own experience as a person who stutters. Like most people who stutter he was baffled by his stuttering. He spent hours trying to figure out what he was doing that made him stutter. He said he felt like a cat in a puzzle box. He finally decided that what he was doing was stopping himself. He said if you want to stop yourself from saying a word, there are three ways you can do it. You can repeat the first sound of the word. You can prolong the first sound. Or you can stop completely. So the question was, why was he stopping himself? When he thought about this, he came to the rather surprising conclusion that the reason he was stopping himself was that he was afraid he was going to stutter. So stuttering, he thought, was nothing but what people who stutter do in an effort to keep from stuttering. It was caused by the anticipation of stuttering. He called it an anticipatory avoidance reaction. And that was the concept that he was trying to verify in a series of investigations that he called studies in the psychology of stuttering.

One logical place to start was with the relation between anticipation and stuttering. For purposes of research, he defined anticipation as the subjects' ability to predict the occurrence of stuttering blocks during oral reading by raising a hand as a signal that they were about to stutter. The relationship between prediction and occurrence of stuttering turned out to be extremely high. There were exceptions. Occasionally stuttering seemed to happen without anticipation as defined in the study. Johnson thought that anticipation of stuttering could occur on a low level of consciousness.

Many of the most basic things we know about stuttering as a response emerged from Johnson's work in the short interval between 1936 and 1938. Chief among them were the well-known adaptation and consistency effects that he demonstrated in collaboration with John Knott. Adaptation became important later when some learning theorists interpreted it for a time as the experimental extinction of stuttering as a learned response. The consistency effect has far more compelling implications. To find that stuttering tends to occur on the same words in repeated readings of a passage means that, as Johnson put it, stuttering is not a random, haphazard phenomenon, but a definite response to identifiable stimuli. What makes the consistency effect particularly significant is the fact that the words that people consistently stutter on tend to be different from subject to subject. Hardly anything could point more clearly to the role that past experiences play in the individual's acquisition of difficulty with specific words. Stuttering is learned behavior, Johnson said, and he repeated it again and again. It virtually became his mantra.

If stuttering is learned, it should be subject to conditioning. Johnson showed that it was. He gave subjects a passage with a red border to read in front of an audience, where their stuttering was relatively severe. Afterward they tended to stutter more whenever their reading passage had a red border, even when reading to a single listener. In the same way, subjects were conditioned to stutter in response to other neutral stimuli such as diagonal lines drawn through words. In a related study, Johnson demonstrated that cues that were associated with past stuttering had a tendency to bring about further difficulty. He blotted out the words that subjects had stuttered in several readings of a passage. When he gave the subjects the passage to read again, they tended to stutter on words adjacent to the blots.

Of course, under ordinary conditions the cues that precipitate stuttering do not take the form of red borders or blotted words. So what form do they take? In oral reading, the cues are obviously words or attributes of words. So the question was, what kinds of words are stuttered? Under Johnson's direction, Spencer Brown did an extensive study in which he noted the stuttered words during many hours of oral reading by adults who stutter. From these data there emerged four factors that appeared to influence the locations of stutterings in the speech sequence. One was a phonetic factor. Words beginning with consonants were stuttered more often than words beginning with vowels. This was true for the subjects as a group. But the phonetic factor also had a strong individual aspect: people who stuttered often tended to have particular difficulty with one or more initial sounds, but these differed from subject to subject. Second, there was a grammatical factor. Content words—nouns, verbs, adjectives, and adverbs—were stuttered more often than pronouns and function words. A third factor was word length: long words were stuttered more than short ones. And finally there was the factor of word position. Words were stuttered more often at the beginning of the sentence than in other positions. In general, then, the stuttering occurred especially on words that were important for the meaning, stood out conspicuously from the context, were evaluated as difficult to say, or began with the subject's feared sounds. Johnson had little difficulty reconciling these facts with the idea that stuttering was a learned anticipatory avoidance reaction.

Finally, he was led to one of the most salient features of stuttering as a response, its tendency to disappear under so many conditions. In laboratory studies he confirmed that stuttering is reduced or absent with rhythmic speech and other speech patterns. He suggested that under these conditions the subjects were fluent because their attention was distracted from the anticipation of stuttering. But he knew that people who stutter speak normally under many other conditions, many of which seemed to him to be compelling evidence for his view of the stuttering block. Unfortunately, few of these conditions are easily studied in the laboratory. So he envisioned a comprehensive investigation of all the circumstances in which stuttering is reduced or absent by means of interviews and questionnaires and by combing the literature on stuttering. This is the study that I did for my doctoral dissertation. It was, of course, Johnson's research. He framed the question. And it was an integral part of the program of research that he had been pursuing for ten years. When he gave it to me to do he explained that the point of the study was that the scientific investigation of any phenomenon is essentially the study of how it varies.

Most of the conditions that my subjects told me about grouped themselves into four categories. First, there were conditions of reduced communicative pressure or responsibility, such as talking to an infant or a pet, or counting from one to ten, or reading a page backward. Some said they could always ask for something in a store once they had pointed to it, or they could say their name after the listener had read it on a slip of paper. Second, there were many circumstances in which subjects appeared to be fluent because they were distracted from their anticipations of stuttering or briefly forgot that they stuttered, for example in emergency situations, when they were taken off guard by the necessity to speak, when they were acting a part in a play, or when they were imitating another person's manner of speech or adopting any novel speech pattern. A third category consisted of situations in which the cues for stuttering were absent, for example, when the subject was speaking a specific language or was in a specific environment. Some subjects stuttered only at home or only in oral reading. One individual who stuttered severely virtually lived the life of a nomad because he was able to communicate vocally only whenever he established himself in a new town. Finally, people who stutter can be made to speak fluently for intervals of time by convincing them that they will not stutter. Posthypnotic suggestion may bring this about. More often, it happens as a result of a person's strong faith in a therapy.

With my study, Johnson's program of research on the variables to which stuttering is related was largely completed. What had he accomplished? His ultimate aim had been to substantiate his concept of stuttering as an anxious, anticipatory avoidance reaction. Certainly, the research had revealed a great many facts that were consistent with the theory. Anticipations and beliefs appear to play a major role in stuttering. To some, they seem to play a decisive role. But not everyone is convinced of that. Heredity does seem to have something to do with stuttering, contrary to Johnson's insistence that it did not; and to some experts, this suggests a concept of stuttering as a breakdown of neuromuscular coordination rather than a goal-directed reaction of struggle or avoidance. However that may be, the fact remains that Johnson's research taught us most of what we know about the way stuttering varies as a response to stimuli. Most of the work on this vital subject that was done later has consisted only of the confirmation and elaboration of Johnson's findings. Perhaps the only notable exception has been the discovery of the contingent stimulus effect. But it was probably Johnson's view of stuttering as learned behavior that helped prepare the way for the great interest that developed in that effect when it was widely interpreted as an example of operant conditioning.

So what are we to conclude from all this, and what has it got to do with the Tudor study and the subject of ethics in scientific research? The Tudor study was wrong. Nothing we say can change that or excuse it. I am a bit dismayed when I hear that the study is to be understood in the context of the looser ethical standards of Johnson's day. There was no dearth of principled people in the sciences in those days. What we learn from all this is that a person can have a lapse in ethical judgment and still be a gigantic figure. Johnson was that. He taught us some of the most fundamental facts we know about stuttering behavior. He had an ingenious theory of the origin of stuttering that came as close to general acceptance as any theory ever did. He was the first to raise the question of the relationship between early stuttering and normal childhood disfluency, and it is due to him that we are still groping for a way to distinguish between them. In his teaching and writing, he taught us not to let language do our thinking for us. He was, in short, a major influence on the thinking of a generation of speech pathologists. I hope and believe that he will be remembered for what he accomplished long after his moment of ethical blindness has been forgotten.

4

THE TUDOR STUDY AND WENDELL JOHNSON

Ehud Yairi

Mass media publicity since 2001 concerning an experiment (the Tudor Study) conducted in 1939 at the University of Iowa with the aim of studying the effect of verbal labeling on the level of speech fluency in children who stutter and in normally fluent children has stirred strong emotional reactions and heated debates about the merit of the study and especially its ethical aspects. Some publications alleged that the investigator, Mary Tudor, a graduate student in speech pathology and audiology at the University of Iowa, and the director of her thesis, Professor Wendell Johnson, attempted to make normally fluent children become individuals who stutter and that they were actually successful in achieving the goal. Several speech-language pathologists concluded that the study provided the necessary evidence for Johnson's diagnosogenic theory and thus had important clinical implications for the treatment of the disorder in young children. The author of this chapter places the study in historical perspective and challenges the central tenets of criticism regarding the objectives and ethical aspects of the study as well as interpretations of its findings.

The Tudor Study: Appraisal of Science and Ethics

In 1939, Mary Tudor, a graduate student in speech pathology and audiology at the University of Iowa, completed a masters thesis entitled *An Experimental Study of the Effect of Evaluative Labeling on Speech Fluency*. It was designed to test several assumptions related to the power of applying the labels "stuttering" and "normal speaker" on the level of speech disfluency of people who stutter as well as normal speakers. The specific questions, found in page 2 of the thesis, were as follows:

1. "Will 'removing' the label 'stutterer' from those who have been so labeled have any effect on their speech fluency?" In the study, this treatment was applied to five children who stuttered (Group IA). They were told that they did not stutter.

2. "Will endorsement of the label 'stutterer' previously applied to an individual have any effect on his speech fluency?" To answer this question, five children who stuttered (Group IB) were praised for their stuttering.

3. "Will labeling a person, previously regarded as a normal speaker, a 'stutterer' have any effect on his speech fluency?" To answer this question, six normally speaking children (Group IIA) were told that they stutter and should do anything to avoid stuttering.

4. "Will endorsement of the label 'normal speaker' previously applied to an individual have any effect on his speech fluency? Six normally speaking children (Group IIB) were told that their speech was good" (Tudor, 1939, p. 2).

Each child in the four groups had several individual sessions with the experimenter during a period of four to five months. The "treatment" delivered in the study consisted of the experimenter's responses to the child during conversation, attempting to implement the general guidelines for each group. For example, when a child in Group IA talked about his stuttering, the investigator said that the child did not really stutter, and was only repeating words being unsure of what to say. On the other hand, when a child in Group IIA exhibited normal speech disfluency, the experimenter said it was stuttering. The child was advised to stop and say the word over again, take a deep breath when he or she was disfluent, and watch his or her speech all the time and do something about it.

Tudor's thesis was directed by Professor Wendell Johnson, a highly admired figure in the short history of the modern discipline of speech-language pathology and audiology. Known for his many contributions to theory, research, and treatment of stuttering until his death in 1965, his work and ideas continued to exert enormous influence for several decades after his death. Like thousands of other theses and dissertations, the Tudor thesis was (a) duly placed in the University of Iowa library, (b) made available to the public, and (c) checked out and read by a good number of scholars over a long period of time.

Approximately 62 years later on June 11, 2001, the *San Jose Mercury News*, a California newspaper, published an investigative report written by James Dyer that supposedly exposed Tudor's masters thesis as an experimental work that violated basic ethics of research with human beings, alleging that it had been suppressed for six decades from the public. According to Mr. Dyer, the thesis reported an experiment designed to make normally speaking children become individuals who stutter (Group IIA) and was motivated by Johnson's desire to test his famous "diagnosogenic theory." For the benefit of readers who are not versed with the scientific literature about stuttering, the theory's primary tenet was that the mere diagnosis of a young child's speech as "stuttering" could cause the disorder. Johnson and his associates (1959), in a full exposition of their ideas, suggested that negative listeners' reactions, in the form of verbal labeling, to typical, normal, effortless speech disfluencies, such as repetition of syllables or words that can be observed especially in early childhood, were the direct cause of the onset of stuttering in young children. When children receive such negative reactions from parents or others, they respond in a variety of ways designed to be guarded from, and avoid, further disfluencies. Their avoidance attempts, however, create tension that, eventually, turns easy, normal interruptions into effortful, struggled speech that we call stuttering. Hence, to substantiate the theory, the *Mercury News* posed, it was vital at the time to show that such a process of creating stuttering can be demonstrated in laboratory conditions. The *Mercury News* went on to state that the Tudor study successfully achieved its objectives, concluding that, "In the experiment, Tudor had subjected half of the children to criticism to make them self-conscious about their speech, eventually driving most of them to stutter." Going even further in revealing names of living participants in the 1939 study, the paper referred to a 77-year-old woman stating that, "At 15 years of age, Hazel, a normal speaker, was induced to stutter." Making bold claims, the paper concluded that the children developed chronic stuttering that was impossible to reverse, that Johnson had suppressed the existence of that study, and that Ms. Tudor (later Mrs. Jacobson), age 84 when the newspaper article was published, was convinced that her experiment did indeed induce stuttering. Finally, the paper reported that several former subjects pointed out Ms. Tudor, as well as the late Professor Johnson, as responsible for their lifetime of stuttering since then. Although apparently ridden by guilt feelings about her role in the study, Mary Tudor argued that as a graduate student she simply did what she was told to do by her academic advisor, Professor Johnson. It is noteworthy that the sensational character of the *Mercury News* report, which was picked up by many newspapers and radio stations nationwide, was enhanced by the fact that the study was carried out in an Iowa orphanage. Michael Erard (2001), in an article published in *Lingua Franca*, repeated several of the central themes pressed by Dyer, stating in a major subheading that, "Sixty years ago, a speech pathologist attempted to turn children into stutterers."[1] In a story published in the *New York Times Magazine*, Gretchen Reynolds (2003) wrote that, "Wendell Johnson was convinced that stutterers are made, not born. To prove it, he tried to turn a group of orphans into stutterers and then ignored the results." She went on to emphasize that "Johnson, to validate his thesis, needed to design an experiment that induced stuttering." Along these lines, Erard (2001) quoted the opinion of the late Dr. Franklin Silverman that, "Dyer's reporting offered crucial support for Johnson's unpopular ideas." The facts, as we shall see, are quite to the contrary. Had the Tudor thesis been a credible study, it would probably have constituted the very first evidence *against* the theory.

Inasmuch as I was interviewed by Mr. Dyer prior to his writing of the story,[2] I would say at the outset that my reaction to his report in *San Jose Mercury News* has been one of dismay with its presumptuous, irresponsible presentation, as well as skepticism about the author's motive and the fairness in reporting. In my opinion, his article misrepresents the objective of the study (as did Ms. Reynolds' article), shows misunderstanding of its theoretical background at the time and, most importantly, contains misleading, faulty statements in that the Tudor thesis does not contain any outcome that he claims it to have, that is, that normally speaking children were induced to become individuals who stutter. Generally, Mr. Dyer had neither proper academic credentials, nor sufficient acquired knowledge, to evaluate the scientific merit of the study to reach his conclusions. His statements, broadcast on many National Public Radio stations, that the study was characterized by a good design and supported the theory, have no basis by any scientific review standards. Having carefully examined the thesis with my colleague (Ambrose & Yairi, 2002), I would say that the *Mercury News* article was wrong on several fronts. The Tudor investigation lacked important elements in the details of procedures design; was poorly executed; and, contrary to the newspaper's conclusions, yielded negative findings about the effects of all four treatments administered, including negative reactions to speech disfluency. The level of arrogant ignorance contained in the article is clearly seen in its conclusion, already stated above, "In the experiment, Tudor had subjected half of the children to criticism to make them self-conscious about their speech, eventually driving most of them to stutter." Where Mr. Dyer is outright misleading in his statement is by conveniently forgetting that half the subjects (Groups IA and IB), *already* stuttered when they entered the study; they were included in the study because they exhibited stuttering. He is misleading because only one quarter of the participants (Group IIA) were subjected to criticism and also in view of the fact that certainly most of the normally speaking subjects, if any at all, including those in Group IIB, were not driven into stuttering. Such confusion and distortion of the basic facts is difficult to comprehend. As will be shown later, the study failed to produce stuttering in the one group that consisted of normally fluent children who were subjected to criticism. Let me now expand here on several points made above as well as on other related issues.

Personal Motivation?

I am not sure what got Mr. Dyer interested in Wendell Johnson's scientific work, but the motivation behind the particular story appeared questionable from the start. Mr. Dyer contacted me with expressed interest in writing an article about the work of Wendell Johnson for a California newspaper. He began the telephone interview with a few minutes of questioning about Johnson's research and findings concerning the onset of stuttering. Then, in a sudden switch, Mr. Dryer spent the next 30 minutes exclusively on a rather minor item (in my opinion) in Johnson's work, asking about what knowledge and thoughts I had concerning the Tudor study, referring to it as the "Monster Study." (This title was borrowed from a 1988 article by Franklin Silverman in the *Journal of Fluency Disorders* and was also used in the Erard [2001] and Reynolds [2003] articles). Although I opined that it was weak, failed to prove anything, and was probably within its era's ethics of research with human subjects, he pressed his opinion, and that of Ms. Tudor (who later became Mrs. Jacobson), that the experimenters did succeed in changing normally speaking children into individuals who stuttered. He contested my views rather than sought them, as if I were a "hostile witness" who failed to fulfill expectations. Such was the interaction during a second discussion, a few days later, following which I faxed to him additional information concerning opinions (e.g., a few paragraphs from Wingate's 1976 book) that dismissed Johnson's diagnosogeneic theory altogether. I also faxed a few paragraphs from Silverman's book (1996) that are more sympathetic to his view. Mr. Dyer left with me an overall impression of being very opinionated and biased about the topic he was working on and wanting to make more of it than it really was. Indeed, the soon-to-appear article contained only one or two lines from our lengthy discussions and the arguments that I brought against the value of the study. Mr. Dyer's zeal was later recognized as excessive even by the *San Jose Mercury News*; he was dismissed from the newspaper for breaking journalistic ethics in obtaining materials for the story.

Testing a "Theory"

As I see it, Mr. Dyer's story reflects a lack of understanding of relevant historic perspectives and the proper time-frame reference. Thus, it projects late ideas and information as if they were there and available during the late 1930s. Specifically, inasmuch as the Tudor study was to test the validity of Johnson's diagnosogenic theory, as stated in his *Mercury News* story, it is interesting to note that very little of that "theory" existed at the time. One should only consider the fact that the initial, very brief expression (literally a few sentences) of ideas placing the diagnosogenic notion as *the* cause of stuttering, appeared in a scientific article by Johnson in 1942, reporting the findings of his first study on the onset of stuttering, three years *after* the Tudor study was completed. Furthermore, the full exposition of the theory was published much later, a full 20-year period after the completion of the Tudor study (Johnson et al., 1959). It is also logical to assume that the study, which was carried out during the first half of 1939, must have been planned some time ahead of that year, perhaps in 1938. It is relevant to note that, during that period, the prevailing theory of the origins of stuttering at the University of Iowa Stuttering Program attributed the disorder to neurologic abnormalities, especially lack of cerebral dominance, in the regulation of the appropriate musculature during speech. Only four years earlier, in 1934, Johnson was advocating far different ideas about stuttering, which relied exclusively on neurologic perspectives, ideas that had not a shred of commonality with the diagnosogenic notions. The following citation illuminates his early point of view:

> The matter of heredity is of some importance in connection with stuttering . . . This does not mean that stuttering itself is inherited. It means, rather, that a particular type of body make-up is inherited . . . In the stutterer, the two sides of the brain appear to be relatively equal in development. As a result, the two sides of the speech mechanism move independently of each other, and when this happens we see the muscle spasm which is the primary symptom of stuttering. *This means that at its bottom stuttering has a physical basis* (my emphasis).
>
> It is a popular opinion that various psychologic factors may cause stuttering. Overindulgence or excessive sternness on the part of the child's parents, excessive timidity in the child, and the child's tendency to imitate the stuttering of other children are frequently mentioned in this connection. These factors are *not* to be regarded as primary causes of stuttering . . . The more important causes of stuttering are physical in nature. It appears that

abnormal birth conditions are among these; at any rate, a much larger proportion of stutterers report unusual birth conditions than do normal speakers. Among these conditions are prolonged and difficult labor, improper presentation (as birth of a child feet first), cyanosis (blueness of the body), difficulty in initiating breathing, and abnormal formation of the head at birth. Illnesses and injuries, especially head injuries, are important causes of stuttering. Poor nutrition in infancy is important in this connection. Prolonged high fever appears to have a weakening effect on the higher brain levels and is sometimes followed by stuttering . . . Perhaps the most important single cause of stuttering is interference with the development of the child's natural handedness" (Johnson, 1934, pp. 2–6).

He went on with several therapeutic suggestions, saying that:

The parent should allow the child to develop his own natural handedness. Without question, much stuttering could be prevented altogether in this way. Certainly it is often possible to eliminate stuttering in its early stages by proper attention to the child's handedness (pp. 7–8).

To me, this historical account supports a supposition that, in 1938, when the Tudor study was planned, Johnson was just beginning to consider a new approach to understanding stuttering but was far from having developed a firm theory that the erroneous diagnosis of stuttering is the main, if not the only, cause. Indeed, the very brief theoretical introduction to the thesis, containing only 60 words, reflects the state of the art at the time. The introduction, refers to the diagnosis of stuttering as "one of the factors" (Tudor, p. 1) responsible for the development of the disorder, and this too as a possibility. Certainly, there is no evidence for us to assume that, at the time, Johnson thought the study would put the children at risk for chronic stuttering. As I said, it is more reasonable to assume that in 1938 Johnson was just beginning to entertain some of the diagnosogenic ideas and was basically looking at the possibility that listeners' reactions can affect the level of the disfluency, normal or stuttering-like, as clearly conveyed in the language used to lay out the stated objectives for the study. It would have been quite a different situation had Johnson directed the study in 1959, when he was clearly convinced about the cause of stuttering and if he had the intention of creating chronic stuttering. It appears to me that Mr. Dyer followed the confused mindset into which Silverman (1988) fell when he evaluated the Tudor study. Silverman begins his article stating that Wendell Johnson initially proposed the diagnosogenic theory in the early 1940s. He continues, however, with a self-contradiction in suggesting that in order to test the theory the Tudor study was conducted in 1939, that is, a few years *earlier*. Going on, Silverman eventually admits that, "The study was done before he formulated the diagnosogenic (semantogenic) theory" (p. 228). He then, however, repeats an illogical position saying that in 1939, "The Tudor study was a part of a program research in which Wendell Johnson was attempting to assess the validity of certain general semantics formulations" (Johnson, 1946)" (p. 228). It is difficult for me to see how the ideas were tested seven years before they were formulated. In yet another turn that strengthens my view and is most relevant to all the critics of Johnson's research ethics is Silverman's firsthand testimony: "Having been a student and research assistant of Wendell Johnson, I find it unthinkable that he would have conducted such a study after formulating the theory" (p. 228).

Scope of the Study

In my opinion, one of the main weaknesses of the *Mercury News* article, as well as other sources that addressed the Tudor study (e.g., Silverman, 1988), is its limited scope. It focused on only one of the four experimental questions and on only one of the four groups of subjects, the group of normally speaking children who were told that they stutter (Group IIA). By zeroing in on this single question and group, the overall scientific orientation of the study was lost and not accurately presented to the public. The two participating groups of stuttering children whose stuttering was either reinforced or refuted and the group of normally fluent children whose disfluency was reinforced were disregarded by the critics and so was the more general objective and potentially broad theoretical and clinical value of the study in assessing the effect of listeners' reactions on the level of fluency in different groups. That is, what happens when the presence of stuttering is refuted (Group IA), when stuttering is reinforced (Group IB), and when normal disfluency is reinforced (Group IIB)? In these respects, the Tudor study was perhaps the first to look into theoretical and research questions that became highly popular two to four decades later. For example, 24 years later, with the rise in the applications of operant conditioning ideas to stuttering, Shames and Sherrick (1963) theorized that reinforcement of normal disfluency may lead to stuttering, and a good number of investigators (see review by Costello & Ingham, 1984) experimented with reinforcement and punishment of stuttering and normal disfluency). But no attention was given to the results of the Tudor study that concerned the other three groups of children.

Consequent to such overlooking, the whole ethical aspect of the Tudor study was also treated in a very selective, out-of-context manner. No question was raised concerning the ethics of reinforcing the stuttering in children who stutter (Group IB), reinforcing (by approving) normal disfluency in normally speaking children (Group IIB), or telling children who stutter that they really have no problem. To make the point a bit sharper, had Mr. Dyer or others narrowed their assessment of the study exclusively to Group IA, they would have had to state that the purpose of the study was actually to attempt to cure stuttering (by lessening the children's concern about it), not to create it.

Terminology and Objectives

Related to the above, an extremely important aspect of the study and the ensuing debate is the language used in formulating the questions, describing the procedures, and reporting the results. In these respects, all the study's objectives addressed the "level of fluency," (not "stuttering," which is fundamentally different). This was measured by the number of disfluent events. It is essential to understand that (1) not all disfluency is stuttering and (2) there is a difference between having a speaker produce speech that contains stuttering events and creating a speaker who stutters chronically.

The first point is that speech interruptions, or "disfluencies," do not necessarily mean "stuttering." Whereas stuttering reflects a perceptual judgment of quality, disfluency is used for descriptive purposes. A disfluency such as "and-and" uttered casually is likely to be perceived as normal; uttered fast and with tension, it may be perceived as stuttering. Disfluency may be used to describe stuttering, but not the other way around. Disfluency types, such as repetition of an interjection (U'hm), pauses, revision (I like-I mean), syllable or word repetition (a-and; but-but), sound prolongation (a→and), and others, are well-known phenomena in the speech of (probably) all normally speaking people. Some disfluency types, however, are more typical of the speech of normally-speaking people; others are found more often in the speech of people who stutter. All types, even the latter ones, however, are also found in normally speaking people, although in considerable smaller quantities. (For a more comprehensive discussion of this topic, see Yairi & Ambrose, 2005.)

As said above, the four questions for the study, restated at the beginning of this chapter, all address effects of the experimental treatment on the level of "fluency" of the four groups, two composed of children who stutter and two of normally speaking children. The objectives of the study do *not* address "stuttering" per se and certainly do not indicate any intent of creating stuttering. Rather, they focus on measuring the "level of fluency," that is, the changes in the frequency of occurrence of certain types of speech disfluency that were counted in the study: syllable repetitions, word repetitions, phrase repetitions, interjections, and pauses. Again, recall that *all* these disfluencies occur in normal speech and that an increase in disfluent output does not necessarily mean stuttering.

Of all the types counted in the study, however, only syllable repetition is clearly more typical to stuttered speech. Word repetitions, which occur in normal speech, *may* also reflect behavior perceived as stuttering. Specifically, repetitions of short, single-syllable words are also quite typical of stuttering, whereas repetition of multisyllable words is more typical of normal speech. The study, however, did not differentiate between the two classes of words. Interestingly, sound prolongation, the disfluency type unique to stuttered speech, was not tabulated although it was mentioned in the investigator's clinical notes. Two disfluency types that were counted, phrase repetitions and interjections, are typically regarded as normal disfluencies. The study, however, did not differentiate between typical and less typical types of disfluencies. Perhaps there was a reason for this.

Historically, research of disfluent speech began in the early part of the 20th century in studies that used a single participant. In the second quarter of the century investigators increased the scope of the studies to include groups of normally developing preschool children (e.g., Adams, 1932; Fisher, 1932). Although repetitions were observed, they were neither defined, nor differentiated, nor quantified. Larger, quantitative research of disfluencies began at the University of Iowa in the second half of the 1930s in a series of studies of both normally speaking children (e.g., Davis, 1939) and children who stuttered (e.g., Egland, 1938). Although initial information about differences in the speech disfluency of the two classes of children began to emerge at the time Ms. Tudor conducted her study, technical constraints restricted the repertoire of disfluency types analyzed, the data were not sufficiently refined, and there was not a very well-developed taxonomy of disfluency types. Against this background, it is perhaps possible to understand why Tudor appears to be quite confused (although being biased cannot be ruled out) in employing essential terminology in a scientific study. For example, in one place in the thesis, she refers to interjection as a "stuttering phenomenon." Actually, however, interjection is the most common disfluency in the speech of *normally* speaking people and rarely would be perceived as stuttering. Consequent to this confusion and/or carelessness, Tudor, in reporting the results, did not make any distinction between disfluency typical to normal speech and that typical to stuttering. Her references to increase in "interruptions" are also misleading, as they may be interpreted by unsophisticated readers to mean "stuttering."

The Children

As specified above, four small groups of children participated, two composed of children who stuttered and two of normally speaking children. Problems arise from the early stage of the study involving the selection of the 22 child participants, all residents of the Soldiers and Sailors Orphans' Home in Davenport, Iowa. First, the overall prevalence of stuttering in the entire child population of the orphanage from which the groups were selected was 4%. This is at least twice as high as expected for a population of children in age range employed (Craig, Hancock, Tran, Craig, & Peters, 2002),[3] raising the suspicion that, for some reason (e.g., low mental abilities), the children were prone to stuttering. Second, and much more important, five judges rated each child on a 5-point fluency scale with 1 being the lowest degree of fluency and 5 the highest. Naturally, one would expect to find substantial differences between the fluency ratings given to children who stutter and to normally fluent children prior to any experimental treatment. Yet, when Ambrose and Yairi (2002) carefully analyzed the data for each subject, there were almost no differences among the four groups. Furthermore, there was no differentiation between children who stuttered and normally speaking children. Two children in Group IA, classified as stuttering, received high initial fluency ratings of 4 and 4.2, appreciably *better* than any of the normal children in Group IIA. This is a real puzzle that seriously damages the validity of the study. Conversely, none of the subjects in Group IIA, classified as normal speakers, received a high fluency rating. The best rating for the group was only 3.1. Such ratings and the absence of meaningful differences suggests the possibility that a few children placed in the normal group were within the range of stuttering. This suspicion is reinforced by the counting of disfluency events in the children's speech. Thus, subject 11 in group IIA was classified as a normally speaking child and was targeted in the study for treatment aimed at increasing disfluency. Her pretreatment speech analysis, however, indicated a total of nearly 7% stuttering-like disfluencies, including 5.23% part-word repetitions. Typically, such a high percentage signifies the presence of stuttering (3% is regarded as sufficient for suspecting stuttering according to Conture [2001], Van Riper [1982], and Ambrose & Yairi [1999]). Why this subject was assigned to the normally speaking group is difficult to understand. For another child (subject 13) selected for this group, clinical notes taken by Ms. Tudor during the first treatment session state, "I asked him . . . Did you ever catch yourself stuttering? Yes, I think so . . . once in a while. You have a difficult time speaking don't you? Nodded head" (p. 83). The notes also indicate that in the first session he prolonged the "f" in the word "fractions." Although such leading questions make interpretation of the child's responses difficult, keeping him in the normally speaking group was an obvious procedural error. Again, I question the integrity of the study on the grounds of subject selection.

A third important detail that casts a shadow on the study is that the children ranged in age from 5 to 16 years, the mean age being 11 years. Children in Group IIA, the focus of the debate and that of the *Mercury News* article, ranged in age from 5 to 15 years with a mean of 10;6. It has been established that, in the vast majority of cases, stuttering begins before age 6 and mostly before age 4 (e.g., Andrews, 1984; Johnson et al., 1959; Yairi & Ambrose, 2005). Therefore, the claim that stuttering was created in several children in the small Group IIA at a significantly higher age raises a red flag. Even an extremely powerful treatment would have been expected to encounter strong resistance at this higher age. This is certainly so in view of the weakness of the experimental treatment applied, as will be discussed later.

Another relevant aspect is that the IQ level of children was rather depressed with a mean of 85. The mean IQ of Group IIA was 84. It is has been documented that the frequency of disfluency and incidence of stuttering is higher in groups of children at low level of intellectual abilities (Bloodstein, 1995; Otto & Yairi, 1976). A final point about the participant children is that no information is provided in the thesis concerning psychological test results, or any other assessment of the children's emotionality, prior to the study. Inasmuch as the investigator later noticed changes in the emotional reactions of the children resulting from the study, the lack of any pretreatment baseline data for this aspect render such conclusions scientifically meaningless.

Treatment

It is worthwhile to note that, contrary to several publications (e.g., Silverman, 1988), Tudor did not read to each child the formal text of the instructions outlining the specific course of treatment for his or her group, which, for Group IIA, may have sounded a bit strong. (The text for Group IIA can be found on pages 10–11 of the thesis). Instead, the scripts served only as general guidelines. As Tudor (1939) writes, "The language actually used in these statements was modified, of course, so as to make comprehensible to the child with whom the interview was held" (p. 11). From Tudor's notes on her interaction with the children, it appears that that language she employed was milder than the formal text. I think, however, that some external supervision, especially at the initial session or two, and ongoing session-to-session assessment of the actual language employed, could have prevented much of any potential psychologic impact and, of course, much of the criticism.

The amount of experimental treatment, however, was small, inconsistent among groups, and the frequency of sessions far between. Although no accurate account is presented in the thesis, extracting from the text, it is possible to conclude that children in Group IIA were seen 8 to 9 times during the entire 4- to 5-month period of the study; other groups were probably seen for only 3 to 4 sessions. Accordingly, Group IIA, the center of the uproar, received an average of one treatment session every two weeks. Also, the orphanage's staff failed to cooperate, as they had initially agreed, in reinforcing the various treatments given to the respective groups. Although no standards exist for optimal number of treatment sessions necessary for therapeutic success in stuttering, and certainly there is no similar information for inducing permanent stuttering, if at all possible, it would appear to me that for the alleged purpose (according to the Dyer and Reynolds articles) of creating a stuttering disorder, the light, spurious treatment was not likely to have the profound effect of (1) inducing chronic stuttering; (2) with such a phenomenally high rate of success as was later claimed; and (3) in individuals who, except for one, had passed the age when stuttering typically begins. Current knowledge of a strong genetic component to stuttering, based on statistical and biological studies (e.g., Ambrose, Cox, & Yairi [1997]; Riaz, Steinberg, Ahmad, Pluzhnikov, Riazuddin, Cox, et al. [2005]), bringing us closer to identify genes underlying stuttering, strengthens my doubts. In light of these and other developments, such as brain research, insisting that a few sessions with the investigator, separated by weeks, caused stuttering, is not a realistic position. Indeed, as will be discussed in the next section, the treatments failed. What is particularly disturbing from a scientific point of view is the lack of any clear plan or rationale for the number of sessions, intervals between them, overall duration of the program, and systematic quantified data-gathering after each session to chart the subjects' progress.

Findings

Regardless of all other considerations presented above about the biased presentation by the *Mercury News*, the study's objectives, the faults with its design and execution, and the serious confusion with terminology that led to improper handling of the data, perhaps the most telling are the actual findings. The Tudor thesis provides two kinds of pre- and post-treatment quantified data on the effect of the different treatments received by the groups: (1) perceptual rating of the children's overall fluency and (2) counts of the number of disfluencies in the children's recorded speech samples. These are reported separately for each child; group data are not available, and statistical tests for significance of differences are not reported. When Ambrose and Yairi (2002) reanalyzed the data, they entered the individual data from the thesis into a statistical package, organized them into tables, and created graphs to facilitate examination. Statistical analyses were applied, as deemed appropriate. The outcome of their analysis clearly demonstrates that, contrary to Dyer's article in the *Mercury News*, the treatments administered had no significant effect whatsoever.

Regarding the perceptual rating, not only were there no statistically significant differences among the four groups prior to the treatment, for each group there was no meaningful difference between pre- and post-treatment measures, and there were no significant differences among the groups by the end of the study. In Group IIA, the normally speaking children in whom, supposedly, stuttering was induced and remained permanently, instead of the expected worsening in fluency, a few children, as well as the overall group's mean, actually improved their rating by the end of the study. That is, their speech was *more* fluent. Particularly striking is the fact that one subject whose fluency score improved was among those specifically named by the *Mercury News* to have developed chronic stuttering as a result of the study. These quantified data illuminate Dyer's false (in my opinion) conclusions as published in the *Mercury News*. Additionally, the five judges wrote informal comments about the children's speech at the *end* of the experiment. Not a single comment made any mention of stuttering for any of the six children.

Regarding the disfluency data, pre- and post-treatment group means for each disfluency type were calculated by Ambrose and Yairi (2002). Applying statistical tests (analyses of variance) to group data that they derived, the two investigators found no significant differences for the groups' pre- and post-treatment count comparisons for any of the disfluency types used in the study: syllable repetition, word repetition, phrase repetition, interjections, and pauses. Interestingly, the greatest change, although not statistically significant, occurred for interjections, which increased in Group IIA. And, for our purpose, it should be pointed out that of all disfluency types, interjection is regarded as perhaps the most *normal* phenomenon. Again, any conclusion stated or insinuated in the *Mercury News* story, or in any other media source, that stuttering was established as a result of the study is refuted by Tudor's own data. The case of subject 11, a girl in group IIA who was presented as a child in whom stuttering was induced, is a perfect example. As suggested earlier, it is quite possible that she entered the study already having mild stuttering. But her pretreatment syllable repetition had actually *decreased* from 5.23 to 0.72 at the end of the study; her fluency rating remained almost unchanged at 3.02 to 2.92, respectively. How, in the face of these data, can one claim that the experimental treatment induced chronic stuttering? One may argue that syllable repetitions were decreased because this child avoided them. Even if this were true, where is the positive evidence for the emergence of a stuttering disorder? A summary of the fluency ratings and the disfluency count data is presented in Table 4–1. The data are based on Ambrose and Yairi (2002).

Finally, the quantitative results were supplemented with clinical notes taken by the experimenter. Perusing these materials that reflect solely the subjective impressions of an investigator, likely to be somewhat biased in hoping to demonstrate at least a measure of treatment effects, the overall picture is that the main changes for the children in Group IIA involved becoming more self-conscious of their speech, reducing willingness to talk freely, lower verbal output, speaking in shorter utterances, speaking

Table 4-1. Mean Fluency Ratings on a 5-Point Scale by Five Judges and Mean Disfluency Counts (per 100 words) Derived from Children's Speech Samples Before and at the End of the Study for the Four Groups

	Fluency Rating		Syllable Repetitions (per 100 words)	
	Before	End	Before	End
Group IA	3.02	2.92	1.18	0.84
Group IB	2.62	2.80	3.56	2.16
Group IIA	2.83	2.92	1.70	0.76
Group IIB	2.88	2.92	0.49	0.41

Data derived from "Normative data for early childhood stuttering," by N. Ambrose and E. Yairi (2002), *American Journal of Speech-Language Pathology*, 42, 895–909. Reprinted with permission.

more carefully and slowly, and perhaps low self-esteem regarding speaking abilities. Although the children's verbal communication, according to these notes, became more inhibited, and occasional mentions of prolongations are noted in two cases, there is no indication that any child indeed began stuttering. In one case, for example, the child adopted the clinician's language and referred to her disfluencies as stuttering. The clinician's description of the child's speech, however, states that the girl would laugh or cover her mouth when she had interruptions but does not mention stuttered speech. Additionally, in some cases, the experimenter's notations indicate increase in the percent of speech interruptions; this, however, was done without any attempt to differentiate between typically normal interruptions and those that are more typical of stuttering. In any event, the quantitative data do not match these statements. It is very probable, based on the data, that much of the claimed increase was in the form of normal disfluency. Finally in regard to the clinical notes, I would like to emphasize that it was scientifically impossible for Ms. Tudor or others to claim that the study caused, or altered, the amount of verbal output or certain emotional reactions as described above. The simple fact is that she failed to obtain any pretreatment measure of verbal output and emotions for purposes of comparison. No meaningful conclusions can be made. All in all, the various sources of information: quantified data, clinical notes, and the experimenter's summary of each case, provide contradictory information.

Summary

The furor ignited some time ago by James Dyer's story in the *San Jose Mercury News* concerning the Tudor study and Professor Wendell Johnson's role in it was biased both on ethical grounds, charging misuse of humans in research, and on assumed findings of the study. In my opinion, both arguments are weak and, in many respects, faulty and irresponsible. Although one may question some ethical aspects of the study, the story resulted in the unjustified staining of the record and reputation of a deceased person, Wendell Johnson.

Let me first comment on the ethics, starting with a question: Is research concerning the effect of listeners' reactions to speech disfluencies on the level of fluency of school-age children who stutter and normally fluent children appropriate to have been conducted either in 1939 or at the present? Inasmuch as I see both theoretical and clinical usefulness in conducting such research, my answer is positive, provided, of course, that the objective is not to permanently increase the stuttering of those who already stutter nor to create a chronic stuttering disorder in normally speaking children, and there are no *serious* theoretical reasons or research evidence suggesting that such risks exist. Depending very much on the specific procedures employed (e.g., the particular form of disapproval of normal disfluency, and the manner in which it is to be delivered,[4] I believe that an investigation commensurate with these objectives, although not just a "fly through," stands a reasonable chance of being approved by committees designated to evaluate research proposals dealing with human subjects.

Indeed, a review of the scientific literature reveals many past studies conducted with people who stutter and normally fluent speakers in which various factors assumed to have the potential of increasing speech disfluencies, at least according to the diagnosogenic theory, were tested. This is reflected in the title of a 1966 scientific article by Siegel and Martin that plainly stated, "Punishment of Disfluencies in Normal Speakers." Although these studies often showed that punishment resulted in decreased stuttering, they were conducted in a period when, according to another article by Siegel (1970), "A frequent observation about stuttering is that it increases and becomes more severe as 'penalty' or punishment for stuttering is increased" (p. 677). A good example is an investigation by Cooper, Cady, and Robbins (1970) on the effects of verbal reinforcement and punishment of disfluencies of individuals who stutter and normally speaking people where disfluencies of both groups were labeled by the experimenters as "wrong" or "right." Daly and Kimbarow (1978) replicated the study with subjects aged 6 to 18 years. Starkweather and Lucker (1978) gave tokens, exchangeable for candy or other items, each time a child stuttered. Some investigators, among them Martin and Siegel (1966), applied electrical shock after moments of stuttering. Lee (1951) reported eliciting stuttering from normally fluent speakers by means of delayed auditory feedback. No one has questioned the ethics of these experiments, and no one has questioned the part of the Tudor study that was designed to see if endorsing the label would increase stuttering in children who were already stuttering. It would appear that making an existing disorder permanently worse would be unacceptable, just as creating new cases of stuttering, were it not for the assumption that the intended and expected increase is temporary.

Taking this view, and with literature evidence cited above, the reader is directed to consider again the rather early, loose diagnosogenic ideas in 1939. The fact is that the Tudor study sought to evaluate effects of labeling on the level of fluency, *not* to create stuttering. Certainly there was no intention of creating individuals who stutter. In this respect, also recall my comments about the broad scope of the study which included several groups, not just normally fluent children, and the discussion of the terminology issue where I distinguished between disfluency and stuttering. Furthermore, even if the study's objective was to increase disfluency to the level that some of it is perceived as stuttering events, it would have been a far cry from anything aimed at making the children stutter chronically. As discussed above, other investigators attempted to *temporarily* increase stuttering in those who already stuttered, and even elicit it from normal speakers. There is no indication that either Ms. Tudor or Professor Johnson believed that, if successful, the study would turn normally speaking children into individuals who stuttered chronically. Considering all the above and the research standards in 1939, ethical criticism of the Tudor study is limited to the failure of the investigators to disclose the purpose of the study to the orphanage's administrator. This is especially true because no parental permission was required and only they (the staff) were in a position to evaluate potential risks and, if necessary, protect the children from potential harm. There was not an informed consent. Also, more external, as well as experimenters' monitoring of the administration of the treatment would have been highly desirable.

Another ethical issue is the tendency in the media and among speech-language pathologists to direct suggestions of unethical conduct to Professor Johnson. Obviously, it was Ms. Tudor who conducted the study from beginning to end for several months, she had the assistance of several people who were knowingly involved (e.g., the judges who rated the children), and she had the orphanage's staff consent for the conduct of the study (but without asking basic questions) as well as for participating in its execution. Why, then, is there a double standard? I do not intend to assign blame. But, if there is blame to assign, then all the above should have been included as guilty parties. Unfortunately, Ms. Tudor (Jacobson) reportedly told Mr. Dyer in her interview that she did what she was told to do by her advisor, Professor Johnson. This is a weak argument that has not been acceptable in much more difficult situations, such as in war. An important lesson for graduate students is that they should not, and cannot, hide behind the back of academic advisors. Students who conduct research share responsibility for the ethics of their studies. A final point about ethics applies to Mr. Dyer and the *San Jose Mercury News*. Mr. Dyer, not being equipped to evaluate the study, provided former subjects with information about the study's purposes and results that, by-and-large were wrong, and only stirred unnecessary agony. Also, by revealing former subjects' names and numbers, additional private information about them that can be found in the thesis (e.g., their IQ scores) was compromised.

Turning to the study itself, as analyzed and discussed above and in much more detail in Ambrose and Yairi (2002), although the basic group comparison structure was reasonable, it was plagued by many other errors in design, execution, data analysis, reporting of findings, and interpretation. Serious questions were raised about the sample of the participants:

1. the unusually high level of stuttering in the population from which the groups were selected,

2. inclusion of many children having low IQ level,

3. inclusion of subjects suspected of exhibiting some stuttering, based on either their own reports or on objective data, in the group of normally fluent children targeted for increasing their disfluency,

4. inclusion of children who stuttered but were rated higher on the fluency scale than normally speaking children,

5. failure to establish acceptable pretreatment distinction among the four groups,

6. unclear, and apparently inconsistent, number of treatment sessions for the different groups,

7. relatively few and far-between treatment sessions,

8. failure to employ any measure to track subject progress throughout the study and assess the language-manner used in implementing the respective procedures,

9. failure of the Institute's staff to conduct follow-ups with the treatment procedures,

10. indiscriminate use of the term "interruptions" as if all are stuttering,

11. indiscriminate usage of the term "stuttering" (e.g., applied to interjections and breathiness in reading),

12. no quantified pre- and post-treatment measure for emotional reactions and speech output, parameters deemed important in evaluating the effects of the treatment,

13. no reliability estimate employed,

14. no statistical tests conducted, and

15. failure of the experimenter to clearly recognize and state that her data did not show any effect of the experimental treatment for any of the four groups.

Overall, this was not a credible study.

Conclusion

Unless additional credible documentation exists to the contrary, the Tudor study must be judged on close scrutiny of the formal thesis document, including the stated objectives, procedures, results, and interpretations. Viewing the total study, in my opinion, reveals reasonable objectives and a reasonable group comparison for testing the effect of positive and negative labeling of speech disfluencies on children who do and do not stutter that, nonetheless, was plagued with numerous critical flaws in its details. A study that, quite certainly, would have been rejected by any reputable scientific journal for its poor quality, was nevertheless exploited by the mass media in ways that have stirred strong emotions and led to unfortunate condemnations.

Based on my review of the historical perspective, the stated goals, and the terminology employed, my most important conclusion is that Wendell Johnson did *not* intend to create stuttering in normally speaking children and certainly there was no intention of creating chronic stuttering as he was accused. In this respect, I would like to repeat my quotation of Silverman, written in 1988, "Having been a student and research assistant of Wendell Johnson, I find it unthinkable that he would have conducted such a study after formulating the theory" (p. 228). Some ethical questions arise, however, concerning the principle of informed consent.

My second important conclusion is that the study failed to show any substantiated experimental effect as outlined in its objectives. It is particularly important to note that it failed to produce stuttering or create individuals who stutter as several articles cited here, as well as others, have claimed. A testimony to this conclusion is Tudor's concluding statement on page 147 of her thesis. It does *not* contain any reference to the post-treatment speech of Group IIA as "stuttering." Perhaps much of the problem with the erroneous interpretations of the study (including those by scholars in the field) can be attributed to the lack of good descriptive data related to disfluency levels and lack of, or lax, taxonomy, which led to some confusion. Some increase in speech interruptions, such as interjections, in some children might not have anything to do with causing actual stuttering. Any other alleged consequences of the study, although possible, have no credible scientific basis that they indeed occurred. Mr. Dyer wrote in the *Mercury News* that sometime *after* the termination of the study a few children in Group IIA began stuttering. Unless these children had already had some tendency to stutter in the past (as suggested by the initial data and descriptions of the children), it would be difficult to explain how the experimental treatment caused stuttering months, or even longer, *after* the conclusion of the study but not at the end of the study as would have been expected. Various developments can unjustifiably, although not necessarily maliciously, be assigned to the wrong agent.

Third, regardless of the state of the diagnosogenic theory in the late 1930s, as noted by Ambrose and Yairi (2002), it has, by and large, been discarded since then due to growing contradictory information and due to the fact that scientific advances link stuttering to strong genetic etiologies. Most recently, Cox et al. (2005) reported findings of the largest linkage analysis of stuttering based on genotyping DNA samples taken from many families of people who stutter. They reported moderate to strong signals for genes underlying stuttering located in a few areas in five chromosomes. Therefore, further attempts to cling to the Tudor study as a proof of the old theory are moot. The theoretical orientation has altered been so drastically that current methods of treating stuttering in young children actually include various ways of calling the child's attention to his/her stuttering, including negative responses to it, by clinicians and parents.

Finally, the repeated assertion that the Tudor Thesis was "hidden" by Johnson is not accurate. Although not published, possibly due to peers' pressure, the thesis has been available to scientists and the public at the University of Iowa Library. Prior to 2001, the year in which the *San Jose Mercury News* published the Dyer article, no fewer than 19 individuals signed their names on the list of readers attached to the thesis. (There may have been other readers who did not sign.) Of these, three read it in 1941, eight in 1942, one in 1946, two in 1951, and one each in 1957, 1983, 1989, 1991, and 1993. The list of readers includes, among others, four persons of whom I have had some personal knowledge: Mary Louis Nelson (1942), Oliver Bloodstein (1957), Marin Young (1957), and Marjorie Goodban (1983). Is it possible that other people who knew about it, for some reason chose to ignore (hide?) it? Unfortunately, Bloodstein, in his *A Handbook on Stuttering* (1995, 5th edition), the most comprehensive text in the field, includes a 100-page reference list but fails to mention the Tudor study.

Acknowledgment

The preparation of this manuscript was partially supported by the National Institutes of Health, National Institute on Deafness and Other Communication Disorders, Grant No. RO1-DC 05210. Principal Investigator: Ehud Yairi. The author's opinions expressed in this manuscript do not reflect the position of NIH.

References

Adams, S. (1932). A study of the growth of language between two and four years. *Journal of Juvenile Research, 16,* 267–277.

Ambrose, N., & Yairi, E. (1999). Normative data for early childhood stuttering. *Journal of Speech, Language, and Hearing Research, 42,* 895–909.

Ambrose, N. J., & Yairi, E. (2002). The Tudor study: Data and ethics. *American Journal of Speech-Language Pathology, 11*(2), 190–203.

Ambrose, N. G., Cox, N. J., & Yairi, E. (1997). The genetic basis of persistence and recovery in stuttering. *Journal of Speech, Language, and Hearing Research, 40,* 567–580.

Andrews, G. (1984). The epidemiology of stuttering. In R. F. Curlee & W. H. Perkins (Eds.), *Nature and treatment of stuttering: New directions* (pp. 1–12). San Diego, CA: College-Hill Press.

Bloodstein, O. (1995). *A handbook on stuttering* (5th ed.). San Diego, CA: Singular Publishing Group, Inc.

Conture, E. G. (2001). *Stuttering: Its nature, diagnosis, and treatment.* Boston: Allyn & Bacon.

Cooper, E., Cady, B., & Robbins, C. (1970). The effect of the verbal stimulus words wrong, right, and tree on the disfluency rates of stutterers and nonstutterers. *Journal of Speech and Hearing Research, 13,* 239–244.

Costello, J., & Ingham, R. (1984). Stuttering as an operant disorder. In R. F. Curlee & W. H. Perkins (Eds.), *Nature and treatment of stuttering: New directions* (pp. 187–313). San Diego: College-Hill Press.

Craig. A, Hancock K, Tran. Y, Craig. M, & Peters, K. (2002). Epidemiology of stuttering in the communication across the entire life span. *Journal of Speech Language and Hearing Research, 45,* 1097–1105.

Cox, N., Roe, C., Suresh, R., Cook, E., Lundstrom, C., Garsten, M., Ezrati, R. Ambrose, N., & Yairi, E. (2005). *Chromosomal signals for genes underlying stuttering.* Presented at the Oxford Disfluency Conference, Oxford University, Oxford, United Kingdom.

Daly, D., & Kimbarow, M. (1978). Stuttering as operant behavior: Effect of the verbal stimuli wrong, right, and tree on the fluency rates of school-age stutterers and nonstutterers. *Journal of Speech and Hearing Research, 21,* 589–597.

Davis, D. (1939). The relation of repetitions in the speech of young children to certain measures of language maturity and situational factors: Part I. *Journal of Speech Disorders, 4,* 303–318.

Egland, G. (1938). *Repetition and prolongation in the speech of stuttering and nonstuttering children.* Unpublished masters thesis, University of Iowa. A condensed version was published In W. Johnson & R. Leutenegger (Eds.) (1956), *Stuttering in children and adults.* Minneapolis: University of Minnesota Press.

Erard, M. (2001). Stutter, memory. *Lingua Franca, 11*(8), 40–49.

Fisher, M. (1932). Language patterns of preschool children. *Experimental Education, 1,* 70–85.

Johnson, W. (1934). Stuttering in the preschool child. *Child Welfare Pamphlets* (No. 37). Iowa City: University of Iowa.

Johnson, W. (1946). *People in quandries.* New York: Harper & Bros.

Johnson, W., et al. (1942). A study of the onset and development of stuttering. *Journal of Speech Disorders, 7,* 251–257.

Johnson, W., and Associates. (1959). *The onset of stuttering.* Minneapolis: University of Minnesota Press.

Lee, B. (1951). Artificial stutter. *Journal of Speech and Hearing Disorders, 16,* 53–55.

Martin, R., & Siegel, G. (1966). The effect of response contingent shock on stuttering. *Journal of Speech and Hearing Research, 9,* 340–352.

Otto, F., & Yairi, E. (1976). A disfluency analysis of Down's syndrome and normal subjects. *Journal of Fluency Disorders, 1,* 26–32.

Reynolds, G. (2003, March 16). The stuttering doctor's "Monster Study." *New York Times Magazine,* 36–39.

Riaz, N., Steinberg, S., Ahmad, J., Pluzhnikov, A., Riazuddin, S., Cox, N. J., et al. (2005). Genomewide significant linkage to stuttering on chromosome 12. *American Journal of Human Genetics, 76,* 647–651.

Shames, G., & Sherrick, C. (1963). A discussion of nonfluency and stuttering as operant behavior. *Journal of Speech and Hearing Disorders, 28,* 3–18.

Siegel, G. (1970). Punishment, stuttering, and disfluency. *Journal of Speech and Hearing Research, 13,* 677–714.

Siegel, G., & Martin, R. (1965). Experimental modification of disfluencies in normal speakers. *Journal of Speech and Hearing Research, 8,* 235–244.

Siegel, G., & Martin, R. (1966). Punishment of disfluencies in normal speakers. *Journal of Speech and Hearing Research, 9,* 208–218.

Silverman F. (1966). *Stuttering and other fluency disorders* (2nd ed.). Long Grove, IL: Waveland Press.

Silverman, F. (1988). The "monster" study. *Journal of Fluency Disorders , 13,* 225–231.

Starkweather, W., & Lucker J. (1978). Tokens for stuttering. *Journal of Fluency Disorders, 3,* 167–180.

Tudor, M. (1939). *An experimental study of the effect of evaluative labeling on speech fluency.* Unpublished master's thesis, University of Iowa, Iowa City, Iowa.

Van Riper, C. (1982). *The nature of stuttering* (2nd ed.). Englewood Cliffs, NJ: Prentice-Hall.

Wingate, M. (1976). *Stuttering theory and treatment.* Boston: Irvington Publishers, Inc.

Yairi, E. & Ambrose, N. (2005). *Early childhood stuttering.* Austin, TX: Pro-Ed.

Endnotes

1. Overall, however, Erard's article is considerably more thoughtful and balanced than other publications.

2. I was also interviewed by Ms. Reynolds as well as by Mr. Erard.

3. The expected prevalence in the population at large is less than 1%.

4. According to Tudor, the formal procedural outlines were applied flexibly to suit the level of each child. Although some examples of the language used in applying the procedure are available, there is no clear description of the actual procedures.

TEACHING RESEARCH ETHICS IN COMMUNICATION DISORDERS PROGRAMS

Barbara Schmidt, Ph.D.
Elizabeth Galletta, Ph.D.
Loraine K. Obler, Ph.D.

The current controversy surrounding the masters level study in which Wendell Johnson guided Mary Tudor in 1939 stimulates consideration of how ethical standards change over time. Not only have ethical standards changed over the 20th century for scientific research, as reviewed elsewhere in this volume (see Chapters 3 and 4), so also have ethical standards in the field of Communication Disorders evolved, alongside the development of knowledge and curricula in the field. In the early 20th century, for example, there was no formal process for peer research review, and the educational requirements in the fields of speech and hearing sciences were rather immature in form. We consider first the development of credentialing and the Code of Ethics within ASHA and then turn to discussion of the ethical issues that confront researchers and educators today in the field of speech, language, and hearing sciences. Then we discuss how research ethics is taught in Communication Disorders programs today, concluding with examples of the formal and informal instruction in ethics at one undergraduate, one masters-level, and one Ph.D.-level program with which we are acquainted.

Development of Credentialing and the Code of Ethics

In the early years of our field, there was no standard professional credential for "speech correctionists" who worked with individuals exhibiting speech disorders. The American Speech-Language-Hearing Association (ASHA), the organization credentialing today's professionals, was established in 1925 with only 22 founding members. It was not until 1930 that ASHA issued its first Code of Ethics, which was part of the Bylaws of the organization. Moreover, it was as recently as 1952 that ASHA issued the first independent document, the ASHA Code of Ethics, outlining the ethical responsibilities of the membership.

Since that first 1952 document, the Code of Ethics has been revised numerous times to reflect changing professional issues. As well, there has been a noticeable evolution in the style of writing used for the Code of Ethics (e.g., Code of Ethics 1969, Section C, (a) "**He** [sic] **must not accept compensation in any form from a manufacturer or a dealer in prosthetic or other devices for recommending any particular product;**" Code of Ethics, 1996, Principle of Ethics III, Rule of Ethics C, "**Individuals shall not misrepresent diagnostic information, services rendered, or products dispensed or engage in any scheme or artifice to defraud in connection with obtaining payment or reimbursement for such services or products.**")

Currently, the ASHA Code of Ethics (2003) identifies four principles of ethics, (see Appendix A for ASHA Code of Ethics, January 2003), which comprise 37 rules of ethics. Only one of those 37 rules overtly mentions students in academic situations directly, and 14 relate explicitly to research and scholarly work. The one rule of ethics making specific reference to students is contained in Principle of Ethics I, Rule of Ethics E and states, "**Individuals who hold the Certificate of Clinical Competence shall not delegate tasks that require the unique skills, knowledge, and judgment that are within the scope of their profession to assistants, technicians, support personnel, students, or any nonprofessionals over whom they have supervisory responsibility . . .** "

The ASHA rules of ethics that relate to research and scholarly work identify eight major issues: (1) discrimination, (2) informed consent, (3) confidentiality, (4) supervision/adequate training of personnel, (5) conflict of interest, (6) accurate dissemination of information, (7) authorship, and (8) plagiarism. Two of the rules—informed consent and supervision—apply most directly to the issues currently debated in the Tudor study. Indeed, the former is a well-elaborated concern for Institutional Review Boards (IRB) in the United States; and, as to the latter, there are unwritten rules, and some written ones, at numerous institutions dealing with ethical conduct between academic faculty and students. Furthermore, despite more rigorous professional efforts to cultivate a culture of ethics in the professions of speech and hearing, the ethical boundaries of research activity remain somewhat vague and might even be considered ambiguous. Although some rules of ethics concerning research appear self-evident, others are more abstract and subject to individual judgment and interpretation. As an example, Principle of Ethics I, Rule of Ethics C states, "**Individuals shall not discriminate in the delivery of professional services or the conduct of research and scholarly activities on the basis of race or ethnicity, gender, age, religion, national origin, sexual orientation, or disability.**" This rule is quite explicit and provides relatively unquestionable guidance with regard to the obligation of the research professional to conduct research without discrimination. In contrast, Principle of Ethics III, Rule B states, "**Individuals shall not participate in professional activities that constitute a conflict of interest.**" Superficially, this rule is clearly stated. However, individuals may perceive a "conflict of interest" differently.

In sum, over the course of the last century as researchers in general have become more concerned with the ethics of our work, the professions of speech, language, and hearing have matured to the extent that there are explicit moral expectations of the members of ASHA. One may well assume that, if the ASHA Ethics Code and the IRB structures were in place today, Johnson and Tudor would have designed and conducted their study differently.

Current Ethical Issues

Even with the evolution of research ethics over the past half-century, and ASHA's Code of Ethics, which attempts to clearly advise professionals of their moral responsibilities, ethical issues in our field continue to require difficult choices. And, although some of the situations involving ethical issues appear rather transparent, even to the most naïve observer (e.g., engaging in invasive surgical treatments as a research protocol without informed consent is clearly unethical), other ethical dilemmas appear more complicated to resolve.

The Tudor study highlights the interplay between teaching, research, and ethical judgment, providing an example of research with multiple layers of ethical issues. In this paper we will focus on three of the ethical issues most pertinent to research. They are: coercion, research methodology, and informed consent.

First, consider the issue of coercion. Coercion should be a basic issue of concern to researchers and professors, as well as students. Typically, coercion conjures up images of vulnerable participants who are at the mercy of the experimenter (e.g., clinical patients who rely on the experimenter for regular therapeutic intervention and thus feel they must participate in research or lose their therapist's goodwill). This is indeed of ethical concern, and the power differential between the researchers and the orphans in the Tudor study today would suggest that particular care be taken in ensuring that the children's participation in the research was voluntary. However, the Tudor study clearly emphasizes the potential for a different form of coercion in a different context as well. In the Tudor study, there was the potential for coercion as a result of the mentor-student relationship.

Typically, mentors are in the position of power vis-à-vis the students they mentor. Presumably, faculty mentors are knowledgeable and have the capacity to guide or otherwise affect the academic progress of a student. In contrast, the student is dependent on the mentor. To avoid compromising the integrity of the educational situation, one might hypothesize that the mentor-student relationship should remain professional and involve a mutual exchange of ideas. We can assume that Dr. Johnson was actively involved in designing the study that Mary Tudor conducted. Mary Tudor was doing a masters thesis project and was implementing the study at the suggestion of her mentor, a professional whom she undoubtedly admired and who was responsible for evaluating her performance. One could hypothesize that, even if she were opposed to the project,

Ms. Tudor might have felt an unspoken pressure from her mentor to implement this study.

In fact, contemplating the past, Mary Tudor questions her own involvement in this study and openly discusses the concerns she had for the children. However, she acknowledges that, as a young student in 1939, she would have been unlikely to challenge the judgment of her mentor (*Houston Chronicle*, 2001). Academic culture in 1939 mandated that students be respectful and compliant to professorial requests. If we assume that students are far less passive in 2005 than they were in 1939, we need to question whether it would be possible for a similar situation to occur today. Indeed, even though current students may be more likely to challenge their mentors, it is likely that we may still find accommodating students, similar to Mary Tudor, who may unwittingly participate in unethical research situations. These students may be reluctant to challenge their mentors and fear repercussions if they do. Or perhaps, student participation in a questionable project might be the product of admiration for a mentor. The extent and nature of the mentor-student relationship may be the determiner.

It has been suggested that a professor-student relationship that becomes a friendship may result in favoritism or exploitation (e.g., Markie, 1990). Students may be selected as research assistants on the basis of a strong personal relationship, rather than on the basis of merit and scholarly interest. Or, self-serving faculty may require students to participate in research projects that are not of theoretical interest to the students, but instead advance the professor's own scholarly work. Favoritism and exploitation of students may be the result of the conscious immorality on the part of professors. Alternatively, professors may themselves be poorly prepared for the ethical dilemmas that research and teaching may present and thus unwittingly make unethical choices. The possible lack of adequate preparation among professors coupled with the expectation that they engage in ongoing research and scholarship may motivate faculty to make poor ethical decisions.

Professors with good intentions, but lacking adequate instruction in research ethics, may entangle students in unethical situations, as Stern and Elliott (1997) point out. As an example, they discuss the issue of deciding authorship, a situation that one would encourage, in principle, during a student-mentor relationship. Stern and Elliot report the case of a medical researcher and a medical student working with the researcher. The student was asked to write a literature review and a preliminary draft of a research study that she had no direct involvement in executing or designing. In return for doing this work, the student would be first author on this publication. Stern and Elliott explain that this medical researcher believed that offering the student first authorship was fair and ethical based on the medical student's valiant efforts on other research projects with less publishable results.

In disagreement, Stern and Elliot argue that, because the student was not directly involved in the study, it was indeed unethical for her to be listed as first author. We would beg to differ, arguing that substantial work can be required to frame a research paper and draw conclusions from its data. Not everyone who works on a given study is involved in each stage of a project (having the idea, designing it, testing participants, coding and scoring the data, running data analyses and statistics, writing it up). For other studies, moreover, these different components of the project demand different degrees of effort. Thus, it would remain an open question what percentage of the work one must do to merit authorship (and who is to judge what work counts as what percent of the total study). Clearly, inadequate ethics preparation of researchers and students alike renders more likely the possibility of making such decisions thoughtlessly.

Second, we should consider the research methodology that is implemented. The Tudor study was designed to investigate the issue of stuttering and develop Wendell Johnson's theoretical framework of the development of stuttering. Mary Tudor labeled children as stutterers over a period of weeks and these children, eager to please the examiner (Mary Tudor), were being reinforced in exhibiting stuttering (i.e., a communication disorder). Clearly, such a methodology would have been outside the boundaries of responsible ethical practice. Encouraging participants on negative behaviors, withholding treatments, administering potentially dangerous treatment are all methodologies that would arouse peer scrutiny today. What Johnson and Tudor did, labeling one subgroup of children as stutterers, even though they were not, would be considered highly problematic today.

Contemporary research protocols in the United States require a researcher to apply for approval to the Institutional Review Board (IRB) in order to initiate a study. This panel of peers (IRB), which is established at any given institution, is responsible for reviewing the research methodology of a study to ensure that ethical standards are maintained. Presumably, were Wendell Johnson and Mary Tudor applying to the IRB for approval to initiate this project today, their research methodology would be challenged. Although researchers are required to obtain approval from the IRB in order to initiate their work, is there the potential for a current masters-level or doctoral-level student in the speech, language, or hearing sciences to participate in a thesis project without obtaining IRB approval? Theoretically, the answer is no. However, it is possible that poorly educated graduate faculty, assuming incorrectly that masters-level "work" is exempt from IRB approval, would not properly educate their students on the need for IRB approval or might permit them to do pilot studies or other work before applying for IRB approval. In such a situation, the system of checks would be circumvented, resulting in ethical misconduct on the part of the student under the direction of the mentor. The result could be the initiation of a research study using an unethical methodology (e.g., withholding treatment without parental knowledge) without the knowledge of more experienced and knowledgeable researchers.

Third, the Tudor study provokes us to think about issues of consent. Clearly, the use of orphans for a research study, as occurred in the Tudor study, raises our concerns about" defenseless" participants. Recall that, the institution that had responsibility for the children in the Tudor study did consent to their participation. But absent a systematic requirement for explaining the risks and benefits of the study, we may wonder whether Mary Tudor or Wendell Johnson advised the institution that these children would be wrongly labeled as stutterers. Furthermore, was it explained that this behavior might be hard to extinguish? These are questions we are unable to answer at this time. However, informed consent in 2005 mandates that the participants, or their guardians, be aware of the details of the study and the potential harm of that study to the participants.

Researchers are responsible for obtaining consent. In obtaining consent, the researcher is responsible for advising the individual of the details of the study (e.g., purpose, method, length of the session, etc.) and ensuring that the individual is not participating under duress. Informed consent should also ensure that the participant is free to withdraw from the study at any point. An essential component in obtaining informed consent is that the individual who is granting consent must possess the capacity to give consent. The administrators of the orphanage were likely to be capable of giving consent on behalf of the orphans. However, was the institution acting ethically when they granted consent? It would appear, at least superficially, that neither the Iowa orphanage nor the researchers were concerned about the ramifications of using these children for this and other research.

In contrast to the apparent lack of concern exhibited by the Iowa orphanage and Wendell Johnson and Mary Tudor about the appearance of using these "defenseless" children for research purposes, current professionals and institutions are concerned about defending themselves against accusations of impropriety during research (O'Neill, 2003). Certainly, appropriate recruitment techniques (e.g., use of letters and flyers, newspaper advertisements, internet lists, etc.), a complete description of the research methodology, and a description of the risks of that methodology ensure the researcher and the participants that appropriate ethical standards have been maintained. However, O'Neill points out that informed consent is possible only if the consenting individual is mentally competent. How do researchers determine if the participant is capable of granting consent? Do researchers assess the adult with an acquired communication disorder for his or her ability to consent? Communication is an integral part of the human self. When communication is compromised in an individual (e.g., he or she has a disorder), the individual becomes susceptible to unethical practices. Is the individual with severe receptive and expressive aphasia and mild cognitive deficits capable of granting consent? Furthermore, does the student researcher, or student research assistant possess adequate skills to make that determination? Moreover, how do we instruct students on these complex issues?

Among other things, consent should prevent deception. In retrospect, we might argue that the Tudor Study involved deception. One subgroup of the participants was labeled as individuals who stutter, a clinical diagnosis with behavioral symptoms.

Therefore, participants were deceived into believing that they had a disorder they did not have at the inception of the study. Some of the children who were involved in this study have argued that this deception had a permanent impact on their lives. Researchers have an obligation in ensure that their work is not deceptive. It is understood that participant bias has the potential to influence the outcome of a study; people who speak freely when they do not think their speech is being examined tend to speak less freely when they know their speech is to be an object of study. Therefore, a researcher may design a study in such a way as to avoid revealing the true intent of the study. However, researchers and IRBs must consider the relative costs and benefits of each instance where even minimal deception is to be employed.

In summary, there is often a complex relation among teaching, research, and ethical judgment. We have identified three of the most salient ethical issues in the work of Johnson and Tudor: (1) coercion, (2) research methodology, and (3) informed consent and reviewed how these issues might be perceived today. Speech, language, and hearing researchers in 2005 are more aware of their moral obligations. However, vigilant attention is required on the part of researchers and educators to ensure adequate knowledge of ethical issues and avoid compromising moral expectations.

Ethics Instruction

The ASHA Code of Ethics (2003) clearly states, "Individuals shall not require (students or professional staff) to conduct research activities that exceed the staff member's competence, level of education, training, and experience" (ASHA Code of Ethics II, Rule of Ethics E). However, no reference is made to the responsibilities of professors who are obliged to educate students on ethical issues. Furthermore, given the reported increase in academic dishonesty (e.g., cheating and plagiarism) in American institutions of higher education (Burnett, 2002; Harding, Carpenter, Montgomery, & Steneck, 2001; McCabe, Trevino, & Klebe, 2002; McMurtry, 2001), it would seem appropriate that members of the academic community aggressively promote integrity in academic and professional behavior.

ASHA has, in fact, established expected learning outcomes for graduate students who study in the speech, language, and hearing professions. Among the learning outcomes cited is the expectation that students will be educated on professional ethics. Therefore, we can assume that ASHA-accredited graduate programs include instruction in ethical issues in their curriculum.

The Council of Academic Programs in Communication Sciences and Disorders (CAPCSD) lists a total of 301 graduate programs in the communication sciences and disorders on their Web site. To explore the emphasis professional training programs place on ethics, we examined the Web sites of 60 of the 301 graduate programs in January, 2004. The Web sites examined were all listed on the CAPCSD graduate program guide and represented programs in 29 different states in the United States. Of the 60 website programs examined, only 9 made any mention of ethics. The mention of ethics in the curriculum of those 9 graduate programs typically appeared in a course description where a general statement was made regarding inclusion of "ethical guidelines" in a course on professional issues.

Because 51 of the 60 programs investigated made no mention of ethics on their Web site curriculum outline, we hypothesize that ethical information is embedded in their general coursework. And, although we would agree that embedding ethics into the coursework is a critical part of instruction, it is important to note that the more explicit the ethical instruction and stated expectations of students are, the more likely students will be to adhere to ethical practices. As an example, McCabe, Trevino, and Klebe (2002) point out that students are less likely to display academic dishonesty in an environment where institutional integrity is a priority. That is to say, if the institution takes a strong position on integrity and enforces a policy against unethical behavior (e.g., cheating and plagiarism), students are less likely to engage in such behavior. We would suggest that this notion should be applied to instruction on professional ethics.

Explicit instruction on ethics in research, as well as in clinical practice, is likely to serve two purposes. First, future professional clinicians and researchers will be cognizant of their moral responsibilities and able to think through ethical dilemmas when they arise or think to ask for help in resolving them. Second, students who continue their education and choose a career in academia will have a foundation in ethics and, therefore, be better prepared to educate their own students.

Therefore, speech, language, and hearing educators need to question the manner in which ethics instruction occurs. Professors need to carefully analyze their expectations of students with regard to ethics. It becomes the obligation of the institution and, therefore, the faculty, to determine if students' familiarity with ethics is sufficient to foster moral decision-making.

"Familiarity" with issues of ethics could mean that an academic program has made a commitment to explicit review and discussion of the ASHA Code of Ethics. This form of instruction would lead to insightful discussion regarding ethical issues. In contrast, however, some institutions or professors have been known to elect to "familiarize" students by handing out the Code of Ethics and suggesting that students review the information contained in the document. Indeed, being handed the Code of Ethics might be construed as providing "familiarity" with the ethical responsibility of members of ASHA. However, this superficial attempt at providing information is not adequate to ensure that students understand the complex ethical issues that may arise in the profession. Given ever-changing cultural mores and the introduction of sophisticated clinical and research instrumentation (e.g., video cameras, voice analysis, Web access, brain imaging, etc.), it is imperative that educators continue to be aware of developments in ethical research practice and be vigilant in instructing students on ethical issues they will need to know, whether or not they themselves are conducting research.

Examples of Ways Ethics Is Taught in Communication Disorders Programs

To understand the range of ways in which ethics is taught at the undergraduate, masters, and doctoral levels, each of the authors reviewed her own program and interviewed colleagues with regard to how they teach research-related ethical issues. All three institutions are located in New York State either near to or in New York City. The programs offer differing levels of academic coursework, thus providing us with perspectives on issues of ethics instruction at the undergraduate, masters, and Ph.D. levels.

Molloy College is in Rockville Centre, New York, which is a suburban area outside New York City. This institution has approximately 2,900 students and offers a variety of majors at the undergraduate level, including a B.S. degree in speech-language pathology and audiology. The undergraduate program at Molloy College has approximately 45 majors at the present time. Though no masters degree in our field is offered, students generally continue on to one elsewhere. The coursework that they take at Molloy is, thus, the students' first exposure to ethics in the context of empirical research and a profession.

At the undergraduate level at Molloy College, all students are instructed on general ethical issues as they relate to society in courses such as "Topics in Social Ethics." Additionally, specialty courses within the major, such as Clinical Practicum and Senior Seminar, focus on clinical and research issues. All Molloy College students, regardless of their major, are required to take a three-credit course in ethics as part of their general educational requirements. Students select their ethics course from an array of possible choices (e.g., Medical Ethics, Communication Ethics, etc.), each intended to familiarize students with moral decision-making within specific life contexts. Although the speech-language pathology/audiology students are not required to take any one specific course in ethics, they are exposed to the notion of moral decision-making. Theoretical discussions often revolve around particular situations and are planned to develop critical-thinking skills. The emphasis is on the larger social ramifications of decision-making. Issues involving a particular profession or research area would be discussed dependent on the perspective of the professor. However, the intent of the requirement is to assist students in understanding the larger implications of moral decision-making, regardless of professional affiliation.

In addition to this general requirement, clinical ethics instruction is explicit in major coursework. For example, issues of ethics are discussed in Evaluation and Treatment Methods in Speech-Language Pathology, a course intended to provide an introduction to diagnostic assessment and treatment protocols. Explicit instruction initially may focus on the need to protect client confidentiality in a clinical setting (e.g., storing records in secure locations, protecting computer passwords, avoiding public discussion of cases, etc.). Implementation of this ethical behavior is carried over into two semesters of Clinical Practicum, the students' introduction into supervised clinical experience. In Clinical Practicum classes, students are advised that a breach of client confidentiality during clinical intervention will result in an automatic failure in the course and may result in a failure to graduate. This policy was initiated by the first author of this chapter in her role as Program Director approximately 10 years ago when it became apparent that a student clinician had acquired historical information about a speech client as a result of discussing the client with a "casual acquaintance" outside the clinical setting. The client who was receiving intervention through the student clinical practicum program was herself an undergraduate student at the college. Prior to the student clinician meeting the client, the author was aware that this client, a student at the college, had had a long history of psychologic problems. As the clinical supervisor, Dr. Schmidt determined that those psychologic problems were not relevant to her speech and language intervention, posed no threat to the student clinician or the integrity of the treatment, and, therefore chose not to share that information with the student clinician. When the student clinician became aware of the client history (as a result of a casual social conversation), she approached the supervisor with the newly acquired information and asserted that she felt she "had a right to know" this information. The professor and undergraduate student discussed the relevance of this information and the manner in which it was acquired. Both agreed that the information had no bearing on the intervention program and that the manner in which the student had gathered this information was completely inappropriate.

In addition to explicit ethical clinical instruction, in this undergraduate program, there is a general introduction into research ethics as well. Each student is required to complete a Senior Seminar course. This course is the capstone course and is intended to provide an introductory research experience. Students complete a research project, which may take a variety of forms (e.g., survey, behavioral observations, meta-analysis, etc.). Margaret Kavanagh, Ed.D., frequently teaches this course. She reports that students receive explicit instruction on ethical issues in research as part of this class. Additionally, she indicates that she meets one-on-one with students throughout the semester to address their individual projects.

Dr. Kavanagh indicates that at these personal meetings she often finds the need to discuss plagiarism, a topic we all note has not usually been sufficiently addressed in more elementary coursework. And, on at least one occasion, it was discovered that students had plagiarized a portion of their senior seminar paper, the culminating activity of the semester. In this situation, Dr. Kavanagh reports that the student was confronted and brought to the Dean for Academic Affairs. The student was assigned a grade of F on that paper and a process of educating the student further on plagiarism and ethics was initiated. In this situation, after careful consideration and numerous meetings with the Dean of Academic Affairs and the professor, the student was given the opportunity to redo the paper and subsequently received a grade of C in the class. Dr. Kavanagh points out that a student in this situation could be expelled; however, to her knowledge this has never occurred.

During the course of our discussion, Dr. Kavanagh was questioned with regard to student projects, consent and approval from the Institutional Review Board. Although she acknowledges the importance of the IRB and the protection it affords participants, she emphasizes that the scope of these one-semester projects is limited and thus far students have not been required to apply to the IRB for approval. Typically, these students do not use human subjects in their research projects. Therefore, IRB approval was not considered obligatory. However, in light of the importance of this matter, she and the other faculty involved in teaching these classes have reopened the discussion of IRB approval for these projects and a new three-credit course will be introduced in the fall 2006 semester in research methodology. This course will facilitate the development of student research projects. The student research projects developed in the fall will be implemented in their Senior Seminar class in the spring semester, thus allowing students the needed time for more implicit instruction on the IRB and submission of an IRB application when appropriate.

In the masters level program in the Communication Disorders (CD) Department at Mercy College students are first educated on ethical issues during an orientation in the department prior to beginning their first semester in the graduate program. During this orientation, the Graduate Admissions Coordinator (the second author of this paper) discusses several policies described in the Mercy College Graduate Handbook as well as policies described in the Graduate Handbook for the CD Department. These policies include descriptions of and actions taken for plagiarism and cheating as well as an in-service on how to use citations appropriately as outlined by the *Publication Manual of the American Psychological Association* (APA). In addition, students are educated on ethical issues in several courses. The two required academic courses that instruct students on ethical issues are Research Methods, a four-credit course, and Professional Issues, a one-credit course. After students have completed these courses, they engage in a research project under faculty mentorship.

In the Research Methods course, students are exposed to ethics that relate to conducting research in the field of Communication Disorders. As a course requirement, students complete the computer-based training offered by the NIH (National Institutes of Health) that educates researchers on the history that led to the formation of Human Subjects protection committees and the formation of Institutional Review Boards (IRBs). After completion of the NIH on-line training, students receive a printed NIH certificate of completion. One faculty member keeps these certificates on file in the Communication Disorders Department.

Throughout the Research Methods course, students participate in a mock-group-research project that involves developing a research question and a research plan. Pairs of students complete the Mercy College IRB application (including an Informed Consent) based on this mock project. For the class discussions, the students are separated into two groups: an IRB and a research team. At the end of the semester, the research team presents the project to the IRB and the IRB questions the members of the research team. Students role-play their assigned title (e.g., chairperson of the IRB, community member on the IRB, Principal Investigator of the research team). This experience (mock project, IRB application, and role-play) allows students the opportunity to run through the research process before they are engaged in student research under faculty mentorship the following semester.

After completion of the Research Methods course, students engage in a research project under the direction of a faculty mentor. This process involves formulating a research question and research plan, completing and submitting an IRB application, obtaining approval from the IRB, testing participants, compiling data, computing statistics, giving a presentation to faculty and invited guests, and submitting a research paper. This research project typically takes students two-to-three semesters to complete. Students are encouraged to submit these papers to a student-poster session at a professional conference, such as the New York State Speech-Language-Hearing Association conference.

In the Professional Issues course at Mercy College, students read and discuss a textbook entitled *Professional Issues in Speech-Language Pathology and Audiology* (Lubinski & Frattali, 2001). The objectives for this course are that students understand issues related to professional education, certification, licensure, standards, ethics, and the profession in other countries. Students are exposed to knowledge of the legislative process with an emphasis on current issues. Topics of discussion include policy and procedures, quality improvement, infection prevention, and professional liability. Current professional issues such as multiculturalism, supervision, autonomy, burnout, and the professional doctorate are also discussed.

In addition to the above-described academic courses, students participate in a clinical seminar course for all semesters that students are enrolled in clinical practicum (typically, this involves three semesters). The clinical practicum seminar courses address ethical issues related specifically to clinical practice. These ethical issues and policies are also written in the CD Departmental Clinic Manual, which is given to students when they are enrolled in clinic. This document discusses both research and clinical issues, and discussing it in class further raises students' awareness of ethical issues that pertain in research.

The Graduate Center of the City University of New York is located in New York City and offers the Ph.D. in Speech and Hearing Sciences. Students in this program typically enter having completed a masters degree in speech-language pathology, audiology, or a related discipline such as linguistics before entering the program. At the doctoral level we focus more on research ethics than on clinical ethics, as our students are virtually all trained and practicing clinicians when they come to us, so our goal is to teach them how to be researchers.

Two topics predominate in our discussions: plagiarism and human-subjects' issues. The first is covered in a couple of pages on "Scientific Integrity" in the school's Student Handbook. In our experience, students do not read that section (or, perhaps, many others) so we include a discussion of plagiarism and the ways to avoid it (appropriate citation, paraphrasing, and note-taking) in our required (but only two credits instead of the usual three) class on Professional Issues (instituted about 5 years ago, taught once every 2 years.). Also, we hold colloquia on the topic every couple of years with catchy titles like "Are you sure you know what counts as plagiarism?" The timing of these tends to be the semester after incidents the faculty are concerned about. Plagiarism (knowing what it is and avoiding it) is also mentioned in the orientation for students, and several years ago we initiated a letter describing what plagiarism is and how to avoid it, which we ask students to read and sign affirming that they have read it, as they enter the program. Students' signed letters are then kept in their files.

Other colloquium topics on ethics issues that have proven necessary are ones on authorship guidelines. In colloquia on getting a job, doing postdoctoral work, and so forth, ethical issues are touched on as well. Among other topics covered in the required Professional Issues class on ethical issues including scientific fraud, appropriate relationships between students and professors, authorship decisions, and so forth. Some professors make a point of bringing up ethical issues in their content classes as well as in laboratory meetings. In a class on Language in Aging and Dementia, for example, the issues concerning how to appropriately obtain informed consent from demented patients or their guardians (although not all demented patients have legally appointed guardians) comes up; whom to involve in signing informed-consent documents; and where one might draw a line between cajoling a participant with dementia to continue testing and coercing him or her to. Similar issues are discussed in the classes and seminars on aphasia, with respect to research participants who have aphasia and, thus, may have difficulty understanding the informed-consent materials and/or indicating verbally their willingness to participate. Analogous issues can arise in classes in research on children.

Another place that educational discussion of ethical issues arises, albeit not systematically, is in the Dissertation Seminar that all students are required to take between the time they pass their Second (focused) Examination and when their dissertation proposal is accepted. These meetings occur once a month; in those meetings students present summaries of their progress in designing their dissertation research and faculty and other students ask questions and make suggestions. Because one of our faculty heads the school's Institutional Review Board, we have quick dissemination in these meetings of the changes that occur over the years in human-subjects regulations at our school. In recent years, for example, it is now considered coercive at our institution to test one's own clients, slowing down the research of some students who choose a particular population to study precisely because it is the population they work with.

In addition, with the NIH requirements that anyone working on a research project pass, now yearly, their Internet-based training on ethical issues in research, students are exposed to the issues covered there at least once in their doctoral training.

Further education, albeit not systematic, concerning ethical issues takes place as specific concerns arise in the program. Once a student sought out another student's scores on the comprehensive examination before they were made available, in order to allay the second student's great concerns; the first student was counseled by the department chair concerning the inappropriate behavior. Other issues have been dealt with more publicly.

When incidents of suspected plagiarism occur, discussion generally only takes place among the faculty. In recent years, these students have been asked to choose to leave the program, but the information about the reason why they left has not been shared with the programs they moved to (of ethical concern for some faculty), nor with the students remaining in the program whose anxiety levels about students "being kicked out of the program for poor performance" have, faculty realized only several years later, been very high as a result. In all such instances, the balance seems to fall on protecting the confidentiality of the accused students involved in such situations. One might argue that this is not ideal for teaching about ethical issues, however, because little information is dispersed. On the other hand, students acquire much knowledge from their classmates during doctoral work, and often such hands-on research knowledge obtained from others in the same research lab is at least as important as what they learn in specific classes or colloquia.

In summary, we were pleased to learn that, at each of our institutions, there is informal as well as formal instruction in research ethics. Understandably, there is relatively more focus on research ethics and less on clinical and student-issue ethics (and those related to students' behaviors such as plagiarism) in programs where students are being trained to conduct research than in programs where that is not the primary focus of their training.

Conclusion

Researchers, professors, and students all have moral responsibilities to the individuals they serve. Ethical conflicts are a part of the student, professor, and researcher experience. As our society becomes more complex, so too do ethical dilemmas become increasingly complicated. It is our expectation that, as the professions of communication (e.g., speech-language pathology, audiology, speech science, etc.) mature, the academic community will further realize the importance of prioritizing ethical education in research and scholarship. As a result, we believe, they will include formal and informal pedagogy concerning ethics pervasively throughout students' programs, thereby fostering professional integrity and competency and yielding better research.

Acknowledgments

We thank our colleagues and students for discussions of the issues raised here over the course of our careers. We are particularly grateful to Professors Margaret Kavanagh, Mira Goral, Gloria Schlisselberg, and Pat Chute for discussions contributing to this chapter.

References

American Speech-Language-Hearing Association. (2002). Ethics in research and professional practice. *ASHA Supplement, 22.*
American Speech-Language-Hearing Association. (2003). Code of ethics (revised). *ASHA Supplement, 23.*

Burnett, S. (2002). Dishonor and distrust. *Community College Week,* *14*(24), 6–9.

Council of Academic Programs. (2005). http://www.capcsd.org/cgi-bin/caplist

Harding, T. S., Carpenter, D. D., Montgomery, S. M., & Steneck, N. H. (2002, November). *The current state of research on academic dishonesty among engineering students.* Paper presented at the ASEE/IEEE Frontiers in Education Conference. Reno, Nevada.

Lubinski, R., & Frattali, C. (Eds.). (2001). *Professional issues in speech-language pathology and audiology.* San Diego, CA: Singular Thomson Learning.

Markie, S. (1990). Professors, students and friendship. In S. M. Cahn (Ed.), *Morality, responsibility and the university: Studies in academic ethics.* Philadelphia: Temple University Press.

McCabe, D., Trevino, L, Klebe, L. (2002). Honesty and honor codes. *Academe, 88*(1), 37–42.

McMurty, K. (2001). E-Cheating: Combating a 21st century challenge. *THE Journal, 29*(4), 36–41.

O'Neill (2003). Some limits of informed consent. *Journal of Medical Ethics, 29*(1), 4–7.

Orphans used in prewar stuttering experiment still suffer effects. (2001, June 14). Houston Chronicle.com

Stern, J., & Elliott, D. (1997). *The ethics of scientific research.* Hanover, NH: University Press of New England.

6

WOULD TODAY'S IRB APPROVE THE TUDOR STUDY?

Ethical Considerations in Conducting Research Involving Children with Communication Disorders

Richard G. Schwartz, Ph.D.

The Tudor Study violated a number of current ethical principles of research with children who were exceptionally vulnerable, given their status as orphans, as children who were institutionalized and communicatively disordered. The study also involved deception and, if the theoretical assumptions of the investigators were correct, put some of the children at risk for emotional distress and for the possibility of developing a communication disorder. Although some general ethical principles may be universal or at least nearly so, most are culturally based and shift with time (generally in the direction of greater awareness and greater restrictiveness). So, in some respects, the study may have reflected acceptable ethical principles of its time. A critical examination of such a study in hindsight remains a useful way of understanding current practice, regulations, and ethics.

Many of these ethical considerations are now codified as part of what is called the Common Rule regulations that govern the research with human participants. They are also codified in the ethics codes of professional organizations such as the American Psychological Association (1992) and, recently, the American Speech-Language-Hearing Association (2003). None of these regulations or codes existed at the time Mary Tudor conducted the research involved in her masters thesis. Nor was the mechanism of the Institutional Review Board (IRB) in place when the study was conducted. However, some of the ethical issues raised by this research could have been considered by Mary Tudor and her advisor, Wendell Johnson. The purpose of this chapter is to consider how today's ethical standards, common research practice, regulations, and professional ethics might be brought to bear on the ethical evaluation of such a study. I will also suggest a form such a study might have to take to conform to current standards. All this will be in service of a discussion of the history of human subject protection, current regulations, and ethical practice in clinical research with children.

First, I should say something about an important issue of terminology. In recent years, the phrase *human subject* has been replaced by the term *human participant* in an effort to avoid objectification of research participants. However, despite the good intentions of such a shift, it obscures the power relationship between a researcher and the participant (Sieber, 1992). This is particularly true in the Tudor study where Wendell Johnson, an already distinguished scholar and respected professor at the University of Iowa, sent a student to an orphanage to conduct this study with children. Ms. Tudor also was in a position of power over the children who participated as an adult authority figure who provided positive and negative comments about the children's speech.

History of Human Subjects Protection

The history of human subject protection has its origins in the ethics of patient treatment. In medical treatment, the Hammurabi code of "First, do no harm" certainly is the beginning of patient welfare concern. In communication disorders, many of the early investigations in the 19th century were single case studies of children by parents who were linguists or studies of adult patients by physicians. Because they were descriptive studies, none involved experimental intervention and were minimally invasive. So, physical harm was not a concern. However, several reports of feral children raised other kinds of issues. These involved mixed attempts to describe a phenomenon, a child raised with limited or absent language input, and the intervention (e.g., Victor, the wild boy of Aveyron; and more recently, Genie). As we have become more aware, these cases raised the potential for conflict between the needs of the child and goals of the researcher.

Current research ethics also have roots in the western philosophy of Kant, who maintained the importance of individual autonomy and the irrelevance of consequences, and John Stuart Mill, who focused on the end result in terms of risks and benefits (Smith, 2000). Current ethical practice draws on both of these traditions.

The experiments conducted by physicians in Nazi Germany brought the world's attention to the safety and well-being of human subjects as never before. Before and during World War II, prisoners in concentration camps were subjected to unnecessary surgery with and without anesthetic. They were exposed to chemicals, intentionally infected with diseases, or immersed in extremely cold water all for the purpose of observing the effects on the prisoners so that the physicians could be prepared to deal with such conditions in German soldiers. These experiments were conducted with complete disregard for welfare of the prisoners who were not told of the risks and had no choice but to participate. The discovery of this experimentation at the end of the war led to the Nuremberg Code, which was developed as the guide for the Nuremberg Military Tribunal. The code set forth standards for research with human subjects. The first basic principle established in the code was the requirement of voluntary consent. The code also stated that subject had to have the capacity to consent, that the consent had to be given without direct or indirect coercion, and that subjects had to be able to comprehend the risks and benefits of the research. Researchers were also required to minimize risk and harm, to establish a ratio of benefit to risk for the subjects that was favorable to the subject, to employ appropriate research designs, and to permit the subject to withdraw from the research at any time.

In 1964, the World Medical Assembly issued The Declaration of Helsinki: Recommendations Guiding Medical Doctors in

Biomedical Research Involving Human Subjects. The recommendations were similar to those made in the Nuremberg Code. The recommendations have been revised twice. The Helsinki Declaration is important because of its distinction between therapeutic and nontherapeutic research and the recognition of the risks involved in nontherapeutic research.

Unfortunately, despite the worldwide attention to these abuses and the guidelines established, abuses have continued (see Sieber, 1992). For example, in the Tuskegee study, African-American men with syphilis were followed to examine the outcome of long-term infection without treatment. This study began in 1932 and did not end until 1972. The most disturbing part of this investigation was that even after penicillin became widely available, the treatment was withheld from these men so that the study of the untreated outcome of syphilis could continue. Other significant violations occurred during the period from 1947 through the 1970s. Among the most often discussed involved the experimentation on patients at the Willowbrook Psychiatric Institute on Long Island, the injection of cancer cells into elderly Jewish patients, the studies in which individuals were deliberately exposed to radiation, the psychedelic drug experiments, and the use of thalidomide. Because these studies are not directly relevant to the type of research that is the focus of this chapter, I will not describe these cases in depth (see Suggested Readings).

These experiments all violated various principles established in the Nuremberg Code and in the Declaration of Helsinki. Consequently, in 1974 Congress enacted the National Research Act, thus establishing the National Commission for the Protection of Human Subjects of Biomedical and Behavioral Research. One significant advance of this act was the inclusion of behavioral research. The Commission identified the basic ethical principles that should underlie biomedical and behavioral research involving human subjects and developed practice guidelines. The Commission considered the distinctions between biomedical and behavioral research and clinical practice, the assessment of risk-benefit criteria in research with human subjects, subject selection, and informed consent.

The result of this commission's deliberations was the *Belmont Report* (1979), named for the conference facility in which the commission met. The *Belmont Report* is divided into three sections. The first sets out the distinction between clinical practice and research. The second section identifies a set of core ethical principles for the conduct of research. The third section defines ethical practice in research.

According to the report, clinical practice has the sole purpose of improving a single patient's condition through diagnosis, preventive treatment, or therapeutic treatment with "a reasonable expectation of success." In contrast, research has the goal of enhancing general knowledge by collecting data, testing one or more hypotheses, and drawing conclusions. It is possible for a clinician to try new or experimental treatments and still have the activity considered as practice if the focus is on the individual patient and the goal is not to advance general knowledge.

The core ethical principles set out in the report are: "respect for persons, beneficence, and justice." *Respect for the persons* is demonstrated by treating individuals as "autonomous agents," meaning that individuals have the right to make decisions about research participation with full information and with freedom from coercion. It also means that individuals whose autonomy is restricted should be protected. Some people's autonomy is constrained because of inherent or acquired characteristics. For example, children, the elderly, women who are pregnant, prisoners, individuals who have diminished abilities to understand what is being asked of them and the consequences of their participation in research all must be treated with extra care. Extra efforts must be made to ensure that these individuals understand as much as they are able about the research and the consequences of their participation. Furthermore, investigators must be aware that the power differential between the investigator and these potential subjects is amplified. In some cases, other individuals responsible for their decision-making (e.g., guardians, parents, etc.) must give their permission. These decision makers must maintain the interest of the individual for whom they are responsible as paramount. In some cases, these individuals are excluded from research.

The second principle, *Beneficence*, refers to the *obligation* of the researcher to not do harm, to maximize possible benefits for the subjects, and to minimize possible harms. Possible harm must be considered in relation to potential benefits. Decisions are more difficult as the risk of harm increases. Although the researcher is responsible for making this determination initially, the researcher is not the best person to make the final decision about the nature, magnitude, and acceptability of the risk.

The final principle stated in the *Belmont Report* is *Justice*. In this case, the word refers to the notion that the benefits and risks of research should be fairly distributed in the population and fairly applied to individuals. For example, until the middle of the 20th century, it was common to recruit subjects from among the poor, the imprisoned, and the disenfranchised. This was the environment and the practice that led to the experiments of Nazi physicians, the Tuskegee syphilis study, and even the Tudor study. This practice was based on the availability, the ease of recruitment, and the powerlessness of such individuals. The research was unrelated to these subjects' racial, socioeconomic, or institutionalized status. The potential justification for including only such subjects is if the research is designed to investigate their status. Thus, their inclusion was unjust.

The remainder of the *Belmont Report* focused on the application of these principles to informed consent, the assessment of risks and benefits, and the recruitment and selection of subjects. Informed consent involves three critical features: information, comprehension, and freedom from coercion (i.e.,"voluntariness") Subjects must be told fully about the procedures, the purpose, the potential risks and benefits, the possibility of alternatives to participation (e.g., alternative treatments), who is conducting the research, and its purpose. Subjects must also be given an opportunity to ask questions and receive answers and must be informed that they can withdraw at any time without negative consequences. There are occasional instances in which subjects may not be given complete information. This can occur only when it is required to conduct the research, when there are no concealed risks that are more than minimal, and when a procedure for debriefing is established. All information must be conveyed in a way that ensures subjects are able to understand fully. Accommodations must be made for immaturity and for disabilities that might impair comprehension. When a parent or guardian is involved, care must be taken to insure that this person acts as agent and as an advocate for the subject. Subjects must be completely free to choose whether to participate or to continue to participate.

Risks and benefits must be assessed in a systematic fashion by the researcher and must be presented to the subject. The risks of research must always be considered in relation to the benefits (risk/benefit ratio).The risks must be equivalent or less than the benefits. Although physical risks are the most obvious, psychologic and social risks must be considered as well.

Finally, the application of justice principle must be reflected in the procedures and criteria established for subject selection. It is not acceptable to study populations of subjects who may be more vulnerable because of their socioeconomic status, institutional status (e.g., prisoners, orphans), or the infirmed, unless their status is relevant to the research question.

The National Research Act (Public Law 93-348), which established the National Commission, also established the structure and mechanism of the Institutional Review Board (IRB). Each institution that conducts behavioral and medical research is required to establish an IRB. The IRB must include nonscientists and one or more members of the community. In many cases, students are also included. The IRB is responsible for reviewing all research involving human subjects before it is conducted. The IRB assesses the ethics of the proposed research focusing on the risk/benefit ratio, the subject selection, and the procedures for informed consent. This legislation also established The Office of Protection from Research Risks as part of the Department of Health and Human Services. This administrative function has now been further separated from National Institutes of Health because of the potential for conflicts of interest. The independent Office of Human Research Protection is now responsible for this function.

Since the National Research Act was passed by Congress in 1979, additional legislation in the 1980s and 1990s (1991) has provided detailed guidelines for the conduct of research and the protection of human subjects. Certain regulations apply directly to research with children and are relevant to our consideration of the Tudor study.

Research with children is specifically addressed in a portion of the regulations adopted in 1983 called Part D (1991). In research involving adults, certain research is classified as exempt (e.g., observation of public behavior, standard educational procedures, surveys, interviews), requiring only approval by the IRB chair or a representative. Research involving risk that is no more than minimal (i.e., no more than one encounters in normal, day-to-day life) can be categorized as expedited and is reviewed by one or more members of the IRB. The final category of research involves the greatest potential risk or populations that are formally or informally considered vulnerable; this type of research is reviewed by the full IRB. For children, research is categorized in the same general way. However, surveys, interviews, or observations involving children can be considered exempt only if the investigator is not involved in the activities being observed.

The issues of risk become even more critical when children are involved. The general principle is that research involving children must have no more than minimal risk to be approved by the IRB. The only exceptions involving greater than minimal risk are cases in which there is likely to be direct benefit for the child or if clinical research will yield critically important generalizable findings concerning the understanding or treatment of the child's disorder with only a small increase over minimal risk. In both cases the experimental procedures must be comparable to those in the child's medical, social, psychologic, or educational experiences.

With the special permission of the OHRP, based on a panel of experts in relevant fields, higher risk research may be approved if the research follows general ethical principles and it provides ". . . a reasonable opportunity to understand, prevent or alleviate a serious problem affecting the health or welfare of children" (PL§46.407).

In all these cases, the researcher must obtain the permission of the parent(s) or guardians and the child's assent. Assent must be obtained in a manner that is appropriate to the children's age, developmental level, and cognitive-linguistic abilities. The researcher can present information to the child orally or in picture form so that a child is able to understand the nature of the research activities. The researcher must also make it clear to the child that he or she can stop at any time without any consequences. The assent can be oral for younger children (under 12 years of age) or in written form for older children. It is possible that assent and the requirement of permission may be modified or waived by the IRB under exceptional circumstances. As in research with adults, the parent or guardian may rescind permission or the child may end his or her participation at any time. Great care must be taken that there is no coercion in the rewards offered for participation. In school-based research, children must be offered alternative activities that offer the same rewards.

Part D strictly prohibits the use of children who are wards of the state or any other institution or agency. The only conditions in which such children can serve as subjects are when the research is related to their status (e.g., a study on the effects of institutionalization on fluency) or if the research subjects are recruited from sites (schools, day camps, hospitals, etc.) where most of the children are not wards. If children who are wards are included in research, an advocate must be appointed for each child who will determine the child's participation and continuation in research. The advocate is an individual with appropriate expertise who is independent of the guardian (or other responsible individuals) and the researcher. The advocate evaluates the child's research participation to ensure that participation is in the best interest of the child.

How Does the Tudor Study Fare in Light of These Guidelines?

The Tudor study fares quite poorly in light of these regulations and guidelines. The ethical deficiencies are surprising even though the study was conducted prior to the existence of the current regulations. There was no IRB or other ethical committee at the time that would have reviewed this research. Thus, the responsibility for determining the ethics of the research rested with the investigators. As mentioned earlier, in the context of the diagnosogenic theory, the negative feedback condition for one group of children who stuttered and one group of children who did not stutter had the potential of serious harm. If the theory were correct, children in the negative feedback condition would develop stuttering. Even if the theory were incorrect, the negative feedback may have caused psychologic distress in the children. There was no potential benefit for the individual subjects. Because of limitations in the design (e.g., number of subjects, pre-/post design) and in the procedures (limited feedback provided only by Ms. Tudor), indirect benefits in terms of a greater understanding of stuttering, improved assessment techniques, or new approaches to remediation were unlikely. The study seems to have design flaws that preclude any advance in knowledge.

These orphaned children should not have been the subjects in this study because the research did not address their institutionalized status. We can only assume that they were chosen because they were convenient and the individuals responsible for their care and welfare apparently were willing to volunteer the children for the study without regard for the potential emotional or speech risks of the negative feedback. It is possible that the institutional guardians were simply unaware of the risk or that they deferred to the investigators from the University of Iowa because of the status of Wendell Johnson or the institution. It seems likely that parents would not have given permission for their children to participate; thus, institutionalized children were chosen. Advocates were not appointed for the children, and the guardians did not act in the children's best interest. According to current regulations this is not acceptable.

The children did not appear to have been informed about the risk and did not appear to have been given a choice about their participation. Because they were not told the purpose of the study and half the subjects were deceived, assent could not have been obtained. There was no planned debriefing, and no provisions were made to ameliorate any of the effects (even those not apparent on the fluency measures) of the intervention.

What Would the IRB Have Approved?

It is possible to imagine a study investigating Johnson's diagnosogenic theory that would be approved by the IRB. The study might take any of several forms. The children would have to be recruited from among the clinical and school populations. Of course, parent permission would have to be obtained along with the child's assent. There is no need or justification for using children who are wards of the state except as they might happen to be attending schools or clinics where the subjects are recruited. The number of subjects and the intervention would have to be sufficient (more than in the Tudor Study) so as to increase the likelihood of an effect of the intervention. A design that is less subject to validity threats than the pretest-posttest design of the Tudor Study would be desirable. Alternatives such as a multiple baseline design or ABA withdrawal designs would be much better ways to examine intervention effects.. The experiment would have to be conducted without the condition of providing negative feedback on speech to stuttering and nonstuttering children because of the potential for harm (increases in disfluency or causing fluent children to stutter), given the assumptions of the theory. Thus, the focus of the study would have to be on the decrease in disfluency in children who stutter by positively characterizing the children's speech and by labeling them as fluent speakers. It seems that this would have to be done by multiple individuals and in multiple contexts for each child. Many other important details would have to be considered by the researchers (e.g., the specific subjects selected, the nature and severity of their fluency disorder, therapy history, whether other therapy would continue). Although this might not be the ideal test of the theory, it would not be possible to include the condition in which children are given negative messages about their fluency status and about their speech, because of the potential harm. Children who stutter would also have to be debriefed in a sensitive fashion because of the inaccuracy of the positive feedback they would be given. One approach could be a period of time following the study in which accurate feedback is given (this could also be a condition in the study). If these children were taken out of therapy or if therapy were suspended for the duration of the study, the researchers would have to find a way to make up this time with sessions in which children receive more generally accepted therapy. If the experimental intervention proves effective in reducing dysfluency, the same intervention should be provided to control subjects.

Conducting Research with Children Who Have Communication Disorders

The general regulations for conducting research with children are the starting point for research involving children with communication disorders. However, some additional considerations are in order. Children with communication disorders and their parents are more vulnerable than typically developing children because of their feelings about the communication disorder. In recruiting subjects for experiments, investigators must be exceptionally clear about the benefits that will accrue to the child and any risks inherent in the research. Some parents may be motivated to give permission because they feel their child will gain some unknown benefit from research participation. Parents must be given a realistic picture of the risks and benefits. Investigators must be sure that assent procedures are presented in a way that is appropriate for children who may have language comprehension deficits.

Great caution must be taken when investigators have a dual role as a clinician and as a researcher. Although dual roles are common in clinical trials conducted in medical settings, special steps must be taken such as consent monitors or separate recruiters and testers to avoid real or perceived coercion.

The vulnerability of these children may be greater than children who are developing typically. Because even young children with communication disorders are aware of their disability, they may be emotionally vulnerable. Various experimental interventions and procedures may have unanticipated effects that need to be considered and either avoided or ameliorated after the fact.

Finally, the use of deception should be limited to cases in which no alternative, nondeceptive method is possible and the deception is justified by the probability that substantive advances in scientific, educational, or clinical values will accrue. Subjects should not be deceived about a significant risk of pain or emotional distress.

Conclusion

The Tudor Study was unfortunate in Tudor and Johnson's lack of regard for the potential harm to the children who participated and in their selection of institutionalized children simply because they were easily available. The deception and the apparent lack of debriefing were also not justifiable. The children had no advocate and were not asked for their assent. Their particularly vulnerable status and the power of the adult researchers from the University of Iowa perhaps should have been considered unacceptable even before today's level of awareness of these issues and the statutory regulation and review processes.

The current awareness of ethical considerations in research involving human subjects, the state and federal regulations that govern such research, the training required for student and faculty researchers, the IRB review process, and the OHRP oversight have created a more widespread awareness of the importance of protecting human subjects. The American Speech-Language-Hearing Association has modified its code of ethics to address human subject issues.

All these factors mitigate the possibility of another Tudor Study. The Tudor Study along with many other unfortunate chapters in research with human subjects during the 20th century have helped us to reach this point. Violations of ethical principles endanger subjects and research endeavors in general because of the resultant loss of public respect and trust of researchers. Furthermore, the findings yielded by unethical studies typically are of little value. Researchers, IRBs, and federal agencies must all remain vigilant to ensure that the rights of human subjects are protected.

Acknowledgment

Preparation of this chapter was supported by grant 5R01-DC 003885 from the NIDCD.

References

American Psychological Association. (1992). Ethical principles of psychologists and code of conduct. *American Psychologist, 47*, 1597.

American Speech-Language Hearing Association. (2003). *Code of ethics.* Rockville, MD: ASHA.

Office for Protection from Research Risks, Protection of Human Subjects. National Commission for the Protection of Human Subjects of Biomedical and Behavioral Research. (1979). *The Belmont Report: Ethical principles and guidelines for the protections of human subjects of research* (GPO Office 887-890). Washington, DC: Government Printing Office.

Office for Protection from Research Risks, Protection of Human Subjects (1991). Protection of human subjects: Title 45. Code of Federal Regulations, Part 46 (GPO 1992 0-307-551). *OPRR Reports*, pp. 4–17.

Sieber, J. (1992). *Planning ethically responsible research.* Newbury Park, CA: Sage Publications.

Smith, M. B. (2000). Moral foundations in research with human participants. In B. D. Sales & S. Folkman (Eds.), *Ethics in research with human participants* (pp. 3–10). Washington, DC: American Psychological Association.

Suggested Readings

Sales, B. D., & Folkman, S. (2000). *Ethics in research with human participants.* Washington, DC: American Psychological Association.

Sieber, J. (1992). *Planning ethically responsible research.* Newbury Park, CA: Sage Publications.

7

SOME PHYSIOLOGICAL STUDIES ON STUTTERING

Katherine S. Harris

This chapter is written in the hope of supplying a little information on the history of physiologic research in speech with, given the topic of the present volume, some notes on the medical and ethical problems that may arise in attempting to do work with such techniques in stuttering research.

Stuttering research is, of course, part of a broad universe of research in applied phonetics; but given this basis, it has not been heavily concentrated on phonetic questions. In Bloodstein's classic text, *A Handbook on Stuttering* (1995), 4 of the 11 chapters are focused on what I would call "state" variables, that is, attempts to identify characteristics of persons who stutter as individuals, such as prevalence and incidence, physiological constitution, personality, developmental history, and home environment. Although such studies are essential, the classification of the individuals as falling within the class of persons who stutter does not tell us much about the stuttering event itself. In general, such studies pose few ethical problems if the subjects' privacy, knowledge of experimental purpose, and consent are adequately guaranteed. My own interest, however, was in concentrating on the utterances of persons who stutter rather than on their characteristics as individuals.

Although acoustic techniques for examining speech sounds are well developed, they do not reveal the movements of the upper articulators, such as the tongue and jaw, the opening and closing movements of the larynx, or the action of the lungs in generating the breath stream. Further, the activity of the individual muscles that generate these movements is not seen. Relatively recently, new techniques have been developed for observing these events. These techniques are of varying degrees of invasiveness and, hence, pose special ethical problems. Somewhat more technical detail on these procedures is given in Borden, Harris, and Raphael (2003).

An Invasive Technique: Electromyographic Research

When I first joined the research team at Haskins Laboratories, we were engaged in establishing the acoustic cues for the speech sounds. We assumed that these cues would be easily segmented out, phone by phone, in the acoustic stream. Because the listener identifies these elements, with only the acoustical signal to work with, presumably its units could be found without a need to refer back to the generating mechanisms of nerves and muscles in the articulators. However, we discovered early in our research that the acoustic signal could not readily be segmented one-to-one to correspond to the units of phonetic description. Instead, the cues for individual speech sounds are smeared into each other, so that the cues for one sound may overlap with those for several others. In an early paper (Cooper, Liberman, Harris, & Grubb, 1958), we suggested that the phonemic invariance might be seen at some level in speech production before acoustic output. In particular, the electromyographic signals for speech sounds might be easier to segment than the acoustic signals. Although MacNeilage (1970) devastatingly and correctly criticized this point of view, it led us to embark on a program of research on the electromyography of speech. In turn, we learned a great deal about muscle function in speech, although the invariance problem is still with us. At the time we became interested in electromyography, it was a well-known medical resource. Electrodes, inserted into a muscle, could, with suitable amplification, record the contractions of individual muscle fibers, or groups of fibers (Harris, 1981). Such recordings were used in the diagnosis of muscle disease, or in describing the function of muscle bundles. The muscles of articulation pose special problems, however. The muscles are small and in general do not lie close to the skin surface; hence, the electrodes must be inserted at some distance from an outside surface.

An essential component in this work was our forming a collaboration with otolaryngologists at the University of Tokyo. This group had developed a technique for recording the electrical signals from the muscles of the larynx, palate, and tongue by inserting electrodes of flexible, fine hooked wires into these articulators, a modification of a technique developed by Basmajian and Stecko (1962). The output signals could be amplified and recorded in parallel with acoustic speech signals. These techniques could be used to answer a number of phonetic questions about, for example, the coordination of the laryngeal muscles in forming voiced and voiceless stops (Harris, 1981) or how the velum is opened and closed to differentiate between nasal and oral stops (Bell-Berti, 1975).

The technique of electromyography also has clinical applications. We could use it to study what happens in a stuttering block. Freeman and Ushijima (1978) examined stuttering blocks in a person with a severe stutter and found that levels of activity in the intrinsic laryngeal muscles during a stuttering block were very high, compared to that of a fluent utterance of the same word (Figure 7–1). Furthermore, the muscles that open and close the larynx may cocontract. Shapiro (1980) found the same results for a small group of adults who stutter severely. However, Armson (1991) repeated the protocol and found neither consistent high levels of activity nor cocontraction of antagonistic laryngeal muscles during stuttering blocks for other speakers. Apparently, there are individual differences among speakers who stutter. As the literature reveals, individual differences are nothing new in the research on stuttering.

However, a number of problems with electromyographic research prevent it from being widely applied. First, it is a difficult

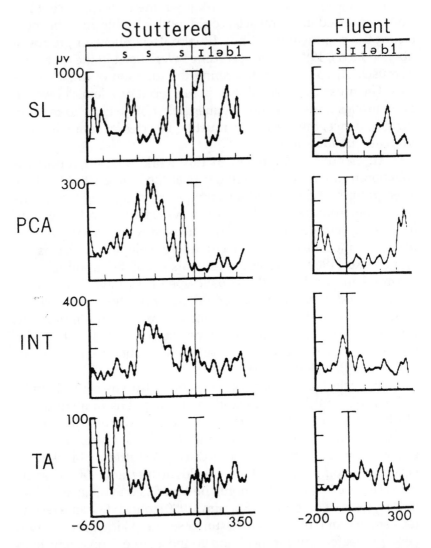

Figure 7–1. Comparison of muscle activity—superior longitudinal (SL), posterior cricoarytenoid (PCA), interarytenoid (INT), and thyro-arytenoid (TA)—for one subject's stuttered and fluent utterances of the word "syllable." (Reproduced from Laryngeal muscle activity during stuttering by F. J. Freeman and T. U. Ushijima. *Speech and Hearing Research*, *21*, 538–562. Copyright 1978 by the American Speech-Language-Hearing Association. Reproduced by permission.)

technique to use. We were fortunate, in the experiments described above, in working with the doctors from Tokyo University Medical School who developed the insertion protocols. Very few American doctors make use of these techniques. Even for the Tokyo group, the "hit rate" for a given muscle is never very high; we were satisfied with about a 50% rate. Furthermore, although the American doctors we consulted were satisfied with the medical safety of electromyography, the insertions are uncomfortable and require a fully cooperative, if not masochistic, subject. This fact excludes the use of child subjects, even if other considerations would not. Our work was almost always done using each other as subjects. Obviously, the number of speech researchers who stutter is quite small. Thus, from the point of view of this book, we are not likely to see an ever-increasing number of speech scientists using electromyography. There was, however, a good reason that we tried it. In the late 1960s, there were very few ways of viewing the articulators in motion. In the last 10 years, technology in the area of viewing hidden body parts has changed. I will mention a study of respiration first and then some use of new techniques.

A Minimally Invasive Technique: Respiratory Research

The techniques for studying the physiologic events associated with respiration in speech have been well researched and have a literature within the field, as pioneered by the well-known work of Hixon (Hixon, 1991; Hixon, Mead, & Goldman, 1976). Although there are differences in technique, the methods for estimating the timing and volume of inspiration and expiration all rest on the fact that when the lungs are filled with air, the chest cavity expands and when the air is expelled, the chest cavity decreases in size. The method of measuring these events depends on estimating the volume of the change. The apparatus for doing so may be a pair of magnets placed on the front and back of the chest wall, whose magnetic output changes with changes in the distance between the magnets or a band wrapped around the chest wall whose output changes with the length of the band when the chest wall expands and contracts. In contrast to electromyography, these techniques do not require penetration of the body surface. They pose no problem or discomfort to the subject beyond the necessity to remain in the same body position through the period of the experiment. Thus, any subject willing or able to sit still is a potential subject, and research is likely to be approved by a Human Subjects Committee.

It has long been known that stuttering tends to occur at the onset of words that begin sentences and even words that begin clauses (Brown, 1937; Quarrington, Conway, & Siegel, 1962). In general, this tendency has been attributed to some characteristic of the nature of the syntactic break itself. Another related possibility is that the association between breath intake and syntactic break is responsible. Of course, these two events are closely related. Speakers, including those who stutter, most often take a breath at syntactic pauses. One may then ask whether the syntactic break or the inspiration is most closely associated with the stuttering event.

I will describe an experiment performed by Russo (2002). She was especially interested in stuttering patterns in young children before these patterns had been altered by therapy. The children were of an age when they were first diagnosed as stuttering, typically at beginning school attendance. Five children were chosen, and age-matched with children with normal fluency. Each child was recorded telling the story of "Goldilocks and the Three Bears" and engaging in a description of a birthday party. During the experiment they wore Respitrace bands (Winkworth, Davis, Adams, & Ellis, 1995; Winkworth, Davis, Ellis, & Adams, 1994). The recordings from the Respitrace bands could be used to locate the onsets of inspiration. An acoustic record was made. The children were seated in a KinderChair to minimize body movement that might contaminate records. The audio records were transcribed, and grammatic boundaries (sentences and clauses) were marked. On this transcript, the position of inspiration onsets was identified. For each child, the temporal positions of non-fluencies were divided into four classes depending on the status of inspiration, and syntax; grammatical boundaries with inspiration, grammatic boundaries without inspiration, nonboundaries with inspiration, and nonboundaries without inspiration. The results are shown for children who stutter and

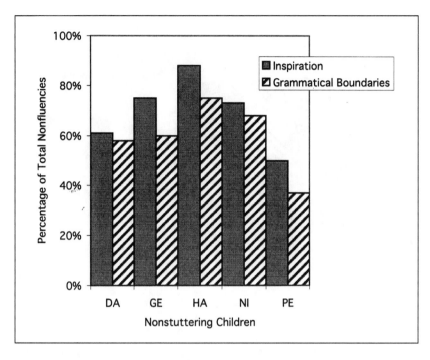

Figure 7–2. Percent of nonfluencies in each of four categories with respect to the onset of inspiration and syntactic boundary for five children with normal speech. (Reproduced from the unpublished doctoral thesis, *Inspiratory placement of young stuttering and nonstuttering children in spontaneous speech*, by A. Russo (2002) at the City University of New York, with the author's permission.)

children who do not in Figures 7–2 and 7–3, respectively. Of course, the children who did not stutter had far fewer disfluencies than those who did; and the total number of disfluencies varied substantially within groups. As we would expect from Brown's (1937) results, for every child, the most stutters or other nonfluencies occur at clause boundaries. Furthermore, we expect, as is confirmed, that inspirations typically occurred at clause boundaries. However, our basic question was whether a stutter was more likely to occur at a clause boundary without an inspiration or at an inspiration without a clause boundary. For each child in both groups, the second class is larger; that is, inspiration

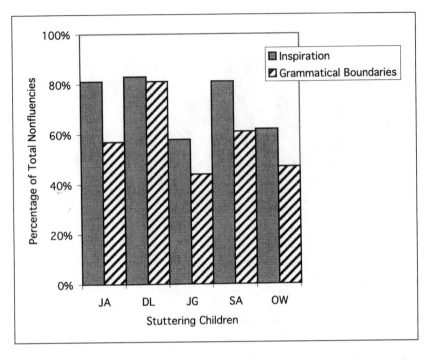

Figure 7–3. Percent of stuttering events in each of four categories with respect to the onset of inspiration and syntactic boundary for five children diagnosed as stuttering. (Reproduced from the unpublished doctoral thesis, *Inspiratory placement of young stuttering and nonstuttering children in spontaneous speech*, by A. Russo (2002) at City University of New York, with permission.)

is a stronger determinant of the presence of a disfluency than is the presence of a clause boundary. This is a result that we could not have obtained without an ability to monitor respiration. The technique has the obvious advantage that it allows us to experiment on a wide range of individuals and gives us information that we could not obtain from the acoustic record. Of course, it is still necessary to obtain the consent of the subject. One little girl in the present study announced after her first session that she "didn't like it here and wanted to go home!" Of course, she was excused from further participation, although she received the same toys as a reward for participation as those who completed the experiment. The other subjects seemed to enjoy the experience.

Minimally Invasive Combined Measures

In the experiment just described, respiration measures showed us when stuttering occurred as a function of syntactic events. In the experiments reported below (Story, 1990; Story, Alfonso, & Harris, 1996), experimental events were examined before and after a well-known therapy regime. The Hollins Precision Fluency Shaping Program (PFSP) (Webster, 1975; 1979) has been shown to reduce stuttering in adults with a long history of nonfluency. Treatment is based on an explicit set of targets, which are taught to the client in a structured program. There are five therapy targets in the Hollins Program:

1. The Stretched Syllable target. The client is expected to prolong syllable duration.

2. The Full Breath target. The client is instructed to take a full breath of air before beginning to speak.

3. The Voice Initiation target. The client is expected to initiate voicing with a gradual onset of phonation.

4. The Slow Change target. The client is expected to make articulator transitions slowly.

5. The Reduced Pressure target. The client is expected to produce voiceless consonants with reduced pressure.

As one can see from the above descriptions, with the exception of the acoustic target in the original program, the subject and the therapist had no way of evaluating the progress of the training, because they had no equipment that would allow them to make physiologic measures.

Four types of measures were made on three subjects who stuttered and who received a conventional PFSP training program. For comparison, the same measures were made on two normal control subjects with no PFSP training before and after the same elapsed time. In each experimental session, the subjects were asked to produce multiple repetitions of, "He see /pit/ again," "He see /pet/ again," "He see /fit/ again," and "He see

/fet/ again," at self-selected slow, medium, and fast rates. The measures were as follows:

1. **Acoustic measures.** A conventional acoustic recording was made.

2. **Respiratory measures.** Measures were made, using Respitrace equipment, of the timing and volume of inspiration and expiration. Using the duration of the acoustic records of the utterances, it was possible to calculate the duration of the expiratory flow.

3. **Laryngeal data.** The movement of the vocal folds was monitored using an optical technique, transillumination. A flexible fiber bundle was inserted into the subject's nose, and positioned just above the larynx. The light from the fiber bundle was used as part of a transillumination system, whereby the amount of light passing through the glottis was sensed by a phototransistor placed on the surface of the neck just below the cricoid cartilage. The amount of light reaching the photocell was used as a measure of glottal opening. This measure has been shown to be highly correlated with measurements of vocal fold separation obtained from frame-by-frame measurement of fiber optic films (Löfqvist & Yoshioka, 1980).

4. **Upper articulator data.** Vertical displacements of upper lip, lower lip, and jaw were monitored using an optical tracking system. Lightweight infrared light-emitting diodes were placed on the middle of the vermilion border of the upper and lower lips and on the jaw midline over the mental protuberance. Light from the diodes was fed to the associated electronics and movement in the y-plane was recorded. The jaw movement was subtracted from the lower lip movement, so the total amplitude of the upper and lower lip excursions could be estimated by summing the two amplitudes. The details of the data collection and analysis can be found in Story's doctoral thesis (Story, 1990), and in the published paper (Story, Alfonso, & Harris, 1996).

The respiratory data are shown in Figure 7–4 (inspiratory data) and Figure 7–5 (expiratory data). The subjects were clearly taking in a larger volume of air after treatment.

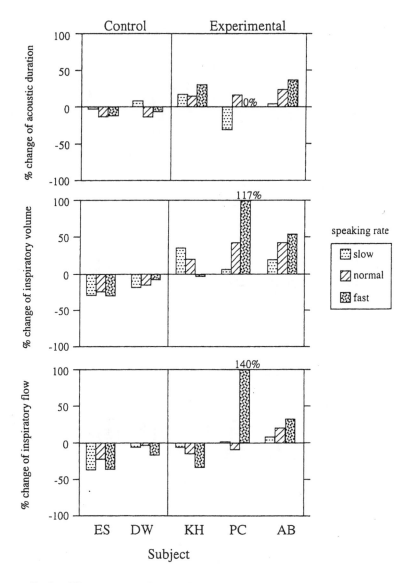

Figure 7–4. The percent change in acoustic duration, inspiratory volume, and inspiratory flow before and after treatment. The change in acoustic duration for Subject PC was too small to indicate on the scale on the graph. "Slow," "normal," and "fast" conditions are indicated by the histogram fill pattern. The subjects are indicated on the abscissa. (Reproduced from Pre- and posttreatment comparison of the kinematics of the fluent speech of persons who stutter by R. S. Story, P. J. Alfonso, and K. S. Harris, *Journal of Speech and Hearing Research, 39,* 991–1005. Copyright 1996 by the American Speech-Language-Hearing Association. Reproduced with permission.)

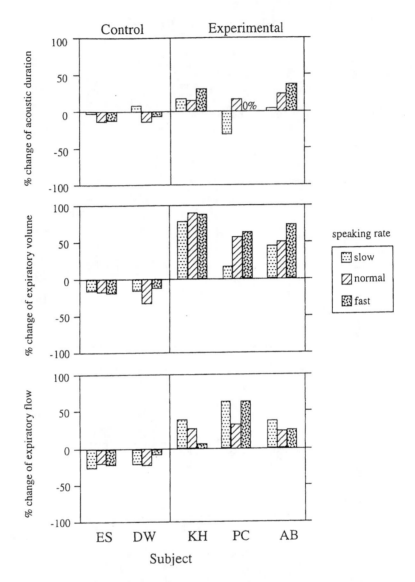

Figure 7–5. The percent change in acoustic duration, expiratory volume, and expiratory flow, before and after treatment. The change in acoustic duration for PC in the fast condition was too small to indicate on the scale on the graph. "Slow," "normal," and "fast" conditions are indicated by the histogram fill pattern. The subjects are indicated on the abscissa. Reproduced from Pre- and posttreatment comparison of the kinematics of the fluent speech of persons who stutter by R. S. Story, P. J. Alfonso, and K. S. Harris, *Journal of Speech and Hearing Research*, *39*, 991–1005. Copyright 1996 by the American Speech-Language-Hearing Association. Reproduced with permission.)

It is possible that this increase in air volume might be a consequence of the "stretched syllable" instruction, rather than the "full breath" instruction, as we know from prior work that subjects tend to take fuller breaths before longer utterances (Gelfer, 1987; Gelfer, Harris, Collier, & Baer, 1983; Winkworth, Davis, Adams, & Ellis, 1995; Winkworth, Davis, Ellis, & Adams, 1994). The results for inspiratory volume and flow are generally opposite for experimental subjects and controls. The controls generally take in less air after the time interval than before. The experimental subjects take in larger amounts of air. Expiratory flow is consistently increased for the experimental subjects after therapy, resulting, probably, in breathier voice quality.

The duration of the laryngeal devoicing gestures is shown in Figure 7–6. Although some values are missing because of technical problems for several cells in the design, we show increases

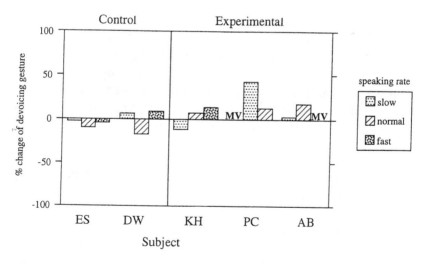

Figure 7–6. The percent change in the duration of the laryngeal devoicing gesture before versus after treatment. Speaking rate condition is indicated by the histogram fill pattern. MV indicates a missing value, due to instrumentation failure. The subjects are indicated on the abscissa. (Reproduced from Pre- and posttreatment comparison of the kinematics of the fluent speech of persons who stutter by R. S. Story, P. J. Alfonso, and K. S. Harris, *Journal of Speech and Hearing Research*, *39*, 991–1005. Copyright 1996 by the American Speech-Language-Hearing Association. Reproduced with permission.)

in duration for seven of nine values for the experimental subjects, but only three are significant. The controls show no consistent pattern. Thus, the result is as we would expect for the Slow Change target, but it is not substantial.

The amplitude of the upper articulator displacement is shown in Figure 7–7. As we would expect, the experimental subjects decreased articulator displacement following therapy, in accord with the Reduced Pressure goal.

Overall, then, subjects did as the therapy instructed, even though they were not able to monitor their own articulation directly. Further support for this notion is lent by the performance of the control subjects. Although the experimental subjects increased in most measures, the control subjects decreased in the same measures.

The experiment shows, I think, that it is possible to obtain information from physiologic studies that is not possible to obtain in any other way. Furthermore, the multiple measures used in this study are not difficult for the subject to tolerate. There is the usual need for the subject to confine him- or herself to an experimental apparatus. A technician of some sort is needed to thread the fiber bundle down the subject's nose and monitor for gagging, but these are not very heavy limitations. Again, subjects must be cooperative, and prepared to sit in a more-or-less fixed position for an hour or two.

Minimally Invasive Measures of Tongue Position Relative to Other Articulators

Thus far, we note that, although accurate ways of monitoring the muscles of articulation, respiration, laryngeal opening, and the movements of the lips and jaw have been developed, the movements of the tongue cannot be described by any of these techniques. Since roughly the turn of the century, steady-state views of the tongue in the oral cavity, as a subject articulated a vowel, for example, have been available. However, it was not until the development of cineradiography that it was possible to monitor such events as the contact and release of the tongue in forming the oral consonants (Kent & Moll, 1972; Moll, 1960). Such techniques were developed at the University of Iowa in the 1960s.

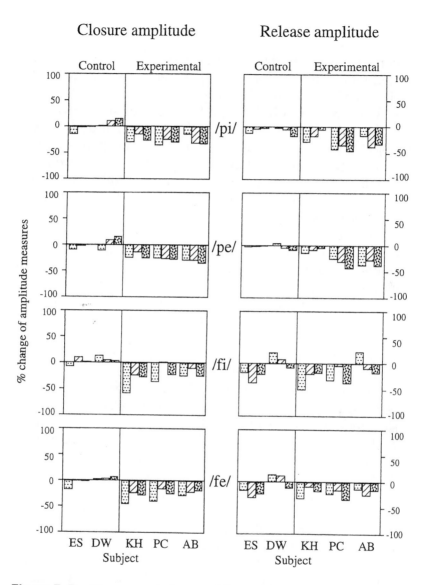

Figure 7–7. The percent change of the amplitude of the closure gesture (*left side of the figure*) and the release gesture (*right side of the figure*) for the target nonsense words /pi/, /pe/, /fi/, and /fe/ before versus after treatment. "Slow," "normal," and "fast" conditions are indicated by the histogram fill pattern. The subjects are indicated on the abscissa. (Reproduced from Pre- and posttreatment comparison of the kinematics of the fluent speech of persons who stutter by R. S. Story, P. J. Alfonso, and K.S. Harris, *Journal of Speech and Hearing Research, 39*, 991–1005. Copyright 1996 by the American Speech-Language-Hearing Association. Reproduced with permission.)

Unfortunately for the development of speech research, however, the techniques used for such an experiment proved to expose the subject to a level of x-ray unacceptable to increasingly cautious Review Boards. To solve this problem, a computer-driven system, the x-ray microbeam was developed which did not expose a subject to the same levels of x-ray, by Osamu Fujimura and his colleagues (Fujimura, Kiritani, & Ishida, 1973) and a prototype was built at the University of Wisconsin. It is still in operation and is currently being used in the study of motor speech disorders by Weismer and Westbury.

More recently, a system was developed by Perkell and his colleagues (Perkell, Cohen, Svirsky, Garabieta, Matthies, & Jackson, 1992). Like the x-ray microbeam, it provides a means for computer-tracking of small pellets glued to the articulators with dental adhesive. However, the tracking is provided by an exterior system of magnetometers, rather than an x-ray apparatus. Because of this difference in underlying mechanism, the system is not thought to put the subject at medical risk. The system is also substantially cheaper to construct and house and is beginning to be commercially available. Such a system is available at Haskins Laboratories and several other speech laboratories. The system requires the subject to sit in a fixed position in a chair.

The experiment described below (Ross, 2000) was designed to examine the well-known effect of increasing fluency in persons who stutter, when various forms of altered auditory feedback are played in their ears as they speak. This phenomenon was studied by examining the fluent utterances of speakers who stutter, as compared with fluent controls, while the movements of the tongue tip, among other articulators, were monitored. The observed movements of the tongue tip for a single utterance sample are shown in Figure 7–8. Two alternative hypotheses about the reasons for the beneficial effects of feedback on the speech of persons who stutter have been advanced. Neither was supported by the results of the experiment. According to "motor control theory," altered auditory feedback is effective by causing subjects to speak either more slowly or less variably. However, neither of these effects was observed for all the subjects who stutter, or under all feedback conditions. A second hypothesis, that persons who stutter have consistent difficulty processing auditory feedback, is not supported either because a given subject

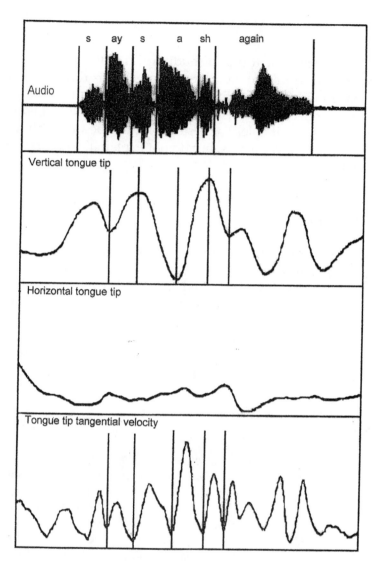

Figure 7–8. Signals for the audio recording with tongue tip signals for a single recording of the utterance "sash." The top panel shows the audio, the lower panels show vertical and horizontal displacements for the tongue tip pellet, while the lowest panel shows tongue tip tangential velocity of the combined horizontal and vertical displacement. Vertical bars show the amplitude of raising for the initial "s," lowering for the vowel "a," raising from "a" to "sh," and lowering to the "a" of "again." (Reproduced with permission, from the unpublished doctoral dissertation, *The effects of auditory feedback on articulation in normal speakers and speakers who stutter,* by D. Ross (2000) at the City University of New York, with permission.)

tends to process all forms of auditory alteration in the same manner, but different subjects who stutter differ in their response mode. Thus, auditory feedback appears to have some nonspecific effect on a given speaker, but the nature of this effect is, as yet, not specifiable. The results of the experiment allow us to discard some hypotheses, but do not explain the nature of the feedback effect.

Conclusion

Looking back over the history of physiologic research on the speech of persons who stutter, we find at least a handful of studies in which the technique used provided either the test of a hypothesis or a demonstration that existing hypotheses were inadequate to explain the observed phenomena. In general, the range of articulatory structures open to examination has increased steadily over the last 40 years, while the discomfort and risk to the participating subjects has steadily decreased.

References

Armson, J. (1991). *A study of laryngeal muscle activity during stuttering episodes: Searching for an invariant physiological correlate.* Unpublished doctoral dissertation, Temple University, Philadelphia, PA.

Basmajian, J. V., & Stecko, G. (1962). A new bipolar indwelling electrode for electromyography. *Journal of Applied Physiology, 17,* 849.

Bell-Berti, F. (1975). Control of pharyngeal cavity size of English voiced and voiceless stops. *Journal of the Acoustical Society of America, 57,* 456–461.

Bloodstein, O. (1995). *A handbook on stuttering* (5th ed.). San Diego: Singular Publishing Group.

Borden G. J., Harris, K. S., & Raphael, L. J. (2003). *Speech science primer* (4th ed.). Baltimore: Lippincott, Williams & Wilkins.

Brown, S. F. (1937). The influence of grammatical function on the incidence of stuttering. *Journal of Speech Disorders, 2,* 207–215.

Cooper, F. S., Liberman, A., Harris, K. S., & Grubb, P. (1958). *Some input-output relationships in speech perception and production.* Paper presented at the Proceedings of the 2nd International Congress of Cybernetics, Namur, Belgium.

Freeman, F. J., & Ushijima T. (1978). Laryngeal activity accompanying stuttering. *Journal of Speech and Hearing Research, 21,* 538–562.

Fujimura, O., Kiritani, S., & Ishida, H. (1973). Computer controlled radiography for observation of movements of articulatory and other human organs. *Computers in Biology and Medicine, 3,* 371–384.

Gelfer, C. E. (1987). *A simultaneous physiological and acoustic study of fundamental frequency declination.* Unpublished doctoral dissertation, City University of New York.

Gelfer, C. W., Harris, K. S., Collier, R., & Baer, T. (1983). Is declination actively controlled? In: I. Titze (Ed.), *Vocal fold physiology: Physiology and biophysics of voice.* Iowa City: Iowa City Press.

Harris, K. S. (1981). Electromyography as a technique for laryngeal investigation. In C. L. Ludlow & M. O. Hart (Eds.), *ASHA Reports: Proceedings of the Conference on the Assessment of Vocal Pathology, 11,* 70–86.

Hixon, T. J. (1991). *Respiratory function in speech and song.* San Diego: Singular Publishing Group.

Hixon, T. J., Mead, J., & Goldman, M. D. (1976). Dynamics of the chest wall during speech production: Function of the chest wall, thorax, rib cage, diaphragm and abdomen. *Journal of Speech and Hearing Research, 19,* 297–356.

Kent, R. D., & Moll, K. L. (1972). Cinefluorographic analysis of selected lingual consonants. *Journal of Speech and Hearing Research, 15,* 453–473.

Löfqvist, A., & Yoshioka, H. (1980). Laryngeal activity in Swedish obstruent clusters. *Journal of the Acoustical Society of America, 68,* 792–801.

MacNeilage, P. (1970). Motor control of serial ordering in speech. *Psychological Review, 77,* 152–196.

Moll, K. (1960). Cinefluorographic techniques in speech research. *Journal of Speech and Hearing Research, 3,* 227–241.

Perkell, J. S., Cohen, M. H., Svirsky, M. A., Matthies, M. L., Garabietta, J., & Jackson, M. T. T. (1992). Electromagnetic mid-sagittal articulometer systems for transducing speech articulatory movements. *Journal of the Acoustical Society of America, 92,* 3078–3096.

Quarrington, B., Conway, J., & Siegel, G. (1962). An experimental study of some properties of stuttered words. *Journal of Speech and Hearing Research, 5,* 387–394.

Ross, D. (2000). *The effects of auditory feedback on articulation in normal speakers and speakers who stutter.* Unpublished doctoral dissertation, City University of New York.

Russo, A. E. (2002). *Inspiratory placement of young stuttering and nonstuttering children during spontaneous speech.* Unpublished doctoral dissertation, City University of New York.

Shapiro, A. I. (1980). An electromyographic analysis of the fluent and dysfluent utterances of several types of stutterers. *Journal of Fluency Disorders, 5,* 203–231.

Story, R. S. (1990). *A pre- and post-therapy comparison of articulatory, respiratory and laryngeal kinematics of stutterers' fluent speech.* Unpublished doctoral dissertation, University of Connecticut, Storrs.

Story, R. S., Alfonso, P. J., & Harris, K. S. (1996). Pre- and post treatment comparison of the kinematics of the fluent speech of persons who stutter. *Journal of Speech and Hearing Research, 39,* 991–1005.

Webster, R. L. (1975). *The precision fluency shaping program: Speech reconstruction for stutterers.* Roanoke, VA: Communications Development Corporation.

Webster, R. L. (1979). *Evaluation of a target based therapy for stutterers.* Roanoke, VA: Communications Development Corporation.

Winkworth, A. L., Davis, P., Adams, R. D., & Ellis, E. (1995). Breathing patterns during spontaneous speech. *Journal of Speech and Hearing Research, 38,* 124–144.

Winkworth, A. L., Davis, P. J., Ellis, E., & Adams, R. D. (1994). Variability and consistency in speech breathing during reading: Lung volumes, speech intensity, and linguistic factors. *Journal of Speech and Hearing Research, 37,* 535–556.

AN ATHEORETICAL DISCIPLINE

Robert Goldfarb

As a rule, all hypothetical constructs tend to fall into one of two broad categories. If they are developed before the facts are in, they are called hypotheses; if they are developed afterward, they are theories (Schiavetti & Metz, 2002). Theories of stuttering, and the challenges to them, are generalizations that attempt to explain a body of evidence following data collection and synthesis. In addition, they may be subjected to future empirical confirmation and may also be considered hypotheses.

Any theory must have two basic qualities. First, it must be parsimonious, or represent the data in a minimal number of terms (Skinner, 1972). Second, it must be falsifiable. That is, the null hypothesis must be taken as a logical alternative to the research hypothesis. In addition, theories or hypotheses, much like politicians or athletes, are given increased status if they can overcome challenges. As more potent challenges are repelled, the theory or politician gains strength. Simply making and verifying predictions are not the best ways to confirm a hypothesis. One also must eliminate alternative hypotheses (Anderson, 1971).

The astrophysicist Stephen Hawking's definition of a good theory is that it describes a large range of phenomena on the basis of a few simple postulates and makes definite predictions that can be tested. "At least that is what is supposed to happen. In practice, people often question the accuracy of the observations and the reliability and moral character of those making the observations" (Hawking, 2001, p. 31).

Myers (1996) bemoaned the paucity of theoretical underpinnings of cluttering, particularly in its relation to stuttering. She noted the interrelations among theory, research, and clinical treatment, surrounding a central definition. Paradigms, which dictate theoretical and research bases of the discipline (Kuhn, 1962), have yet to evolve. Wingate (1977) found that claims of disinterest in theories of stuttering are likely motivated by dismissal of theories that do not relate specifically to a particular therapeutic activity or rejection of challenges to the theoretical base of one's clinical practice.

One purpose of this chapter is to pose and eliminate alternative hypotheses to Johnson's diagnosogenic/semantogenic theory. We can eliminate hypotheses efficiently and convincingly only when they are specified and known. As a generalization of the data dealing with the onset and the moment of stuttering, the diagnosogenic theory is parsimonious and falsifiable. Some of the challenges to the theory lack one or both of these qualities.

Many of the studies below present theories that would be very successful in explaining the onset and/or the moment of stuttering. In fact, it is hard to think of a finding they cannot accommodate. In describing an information-processing theory, Watkins (1981) noted that it "is not only easy to create but, once created, any encounter it may have with data is unlikely to prove fatal." Theories that are not falsifiable are limited both in interest and in usefulness. It might appear that explaining the etiology of stuttering is a choice between poor theories and none. Therefore, much research currently employs an atheoretical approach to the study of stuttering. In reviewing current studies, references made to theoretical constructs may, in most instances, be omitted without obvious loss.

On the other hand, studies without underlying theories may be considered in some ways to be inherently invalid. Construct validity refers to the degree to which a test or measure reflects some theory or explanation of the characteristic to be measured (Schiavetti & Metz, 2002). The test or measure should confirm the theory if the test is valid and the theory is correct. For example, a theory might predict that pathologic and typical participants might use vocabulary with different degrees of fluency. If the test or measure confirmed this, then the measure would have construct validity with respect to that aspect of the theory.

The Causes of Stuttering

Notions of why stuttering begins date from classical antiquity. The Hebrew Bible refers to Moses' halting speech as being "tongue-tied," caused by divine assistance. Pharaoh's advisor suggested a test of intelligence for the infant Moses, who was offered a choice between a bowl of jewels and one of hot coals. If the infant chose the jewels, he was a danger to Pharaoh and had to be killed; the choice of hot coals indicated the infant was not intelligent enough to represent a potential threat. An angel's hand guided the infant's hand to the hot coals. Moses then placed his burning fingers into his mouth causing him to be tongue-tied. The language of scholarly commentary referred to subsequent treatment in terms akin to circumcision.

Other ideas of stuttering as something wrong with the oral structures traced to Demosthenes, who used his famous pebbles to facilitate fluent speech. Aristotle, in ancient times, and Dieffenbach, in 1841, considered stuttering to be the result of pathology in the tongue; the latter performed partial glossectomy as a "cure."

It seems as if nearly every armchair theorist with an agenda has had a turn explaining the etiology of stuttering. Some of the more outrageous concepts included considering stuttering as masochistic behavior, because of the suffering it brings to the speaker, sadistic behavior, because of the suffering it brings to the listener, as well as a particularly bizarre Freudian notion. Here, stuttering is considered a form of anal fixation, where the anal sphincter is metaphorically displaced upward into the oral region and manipulated as stuttering blocks.

One prevalent problem with even the more reasonable ideas about what causes stuttering in the first place, as well as what happens in the moment of stuttering, relates to the post hoc fallacy, more properly, *post hoc ergo propter hoc* (after this, therefore because of this). Put another way, the idea is that if B follows A, then A must be the cause of B. Causal relationships are ascribed to events that may be consequences, as in many of the physiologic studies, or may simply co-occur, as in environmental models.

Some of the models, notions, ideas, and hypotheses follow.

Organismic Models

Nonenvironmental factors are, in some way, causally related to stuttering. *Sex ratio* has been shown to be consistent across the age spectrum (young children, school-age children, adults) and cultures. Generally there are 3 to 4 males for every female who stutters. With regard to *families*, relatives of people who stutter are about 3 to 4 times as likely to have a history of stuttering than are families of people who do not stutter. Among first-degree relatives of people who stutter, the incidence increases. Considering sex of both the person who stutters and first-degree male relatives (fathers, brothers, and sons), incidence is 20%; for first-degree female relatives, 5%. Incidence is higher also in first-degree male relatives of females who stutter. It seems clear that maleness in some way adds to the risk of being a person who stutters. *Hypothesis:* There is a genetically determined threshold for stuttering that is lower in males than females (differential threshold concept). It follows that because males have a greater liability, it takes less in the way of negative environmental factors for this threshold to be crossed. Regarding *twins*, there is concordance (both members stutter) among 78% of identical twins, but only for 9% of fraternal pairs. Yairi and colleagues (Ambrose, Cox, & Yairi, 1997; Yairi, 1997) proposed a hypothesis for a common genetic etiology for persistent and recovered stuttering. Females recover more frequently than males, and recovery does not depend on a genetically milder form of stuttering, with implications for the sex ratio noted above.

People who stutter may be different from those who do not in terms of their *neurophysiologic* structure and/or function. In the 4th century BC, Hippocrates noted that stuttering resulted from accumulation of "black bile." Anomalies have been cited in other structures, including the tongue, hyoid bone, tonsils, uvula, hard palate, and brain. In the 20th century, stuttering was considered a form of aphasia (by Luria) and epilepsy (by West).

Current thinking focuses on subtle differences in the way some of the speech-related neurophysiologic mechanisms seem to function differently for people who do and do not stutter under specific environmental conditions.

Environmental Models

Stuttering can be caused by any of a set of events that lead the individual to believe that speech is difficult, that special precautions need to be taken, and that unusual effort is required to produce it. Differences in prevalence are, at least in part, related to environmental differences, as there are fewer instances of stuttering in permissive and supportive societies (e.g., Ute Native Americans, Malayans, and Polynesians). Stuttering is more likely to be observed in societies where there is marked competition, achievement motivation, conformity, and/or communicative pressure (e.g., Idoma, Ibo, and Kwakiutl peoples).

The strongest environmental theory is *tabula rasa*, or blank slate. Stuttering comes about because speech habits are incorrectly learned or inappropriate attention is paid to the disfluencies that all speakers evidence. *Tabula rasa* may relate both to learning theory and the diagnosogenic theory. However, it is hard to observe antecedent events (the S^D in the operant conditioning paradigm), or to test the notion that the speech of people who stutter is different, at the onset, from those who do not. *Tabula rasa* cannot directly support the diagnosogenic/semantogenic theory.

Interaction Models

Organismic and environmental variables are not seen as mutually exclusive. No organismic variables have been uncovered that are both necessary and sufficient to explain why some people stutter. However the organism is not merely a vehicle to be shaped as a result of the causative relationship between events. Ehud Yairi has received major funding from the National Institute on Deafness and Other Communication Disorders for two projects. The first, comparing children with persistent, chronic stuttering to children with spontaneous remission of stuttering, was funded from 1989 through 2002 (R01-DC000459) (see also Yairi & Ambrose, 1992; Yairi, Ambrose, & Cox, 1996; Yairi, Ambrose, Paden., & Throneburg, 1996). Theoretical models were based on genetic and other epidemiologic aspects of more than 150 children, followed for 6 years following onset. Yairi's grant from NIDCD, on subtypes and associated risk factors in stuttering, runs from 2002 to 2007 (R01-DC005210). It is a multisite project designed to explore epidemiologic, motor, linguistic, and psychosocial factors of stuttering as complex, multilevel, and dynamic processes.

Points of View *(see Bloodstein, 1995)*

1. **The "repressed-need" point of view:** The person who stutters blocks because he unconsciously wishes to block.

2. **The "breakdown" point of view:** Stuttering signifies a temporary failure in the smooth, integrated performance of a complex neuromuscular activity in certain individuals who are emotionally or constitutionally predisposed to such breakdown under conditions of stress.

3. **Biochemical and physiologic theories:** These include the idea of dysphemia, or that stuttering is a mild form of an epileptic seizure (West & Nussbaum, 1929); the report (Freeman & Ushijima, 1978) of a laryngeal component of stuttering; and Schwartz's (1976) description of an uninhibited airway dilatation reflex. According to Bloodstein (1995), there is no conclusive evidence that the average person who stutters exhibits any clinical pathology in these areas.

4. **Neurotic theories:** These include the need for oral gratification, anal gratification, covert expression of hostility, inhibition of threatening feelings and messages, fear of castration, repressed aggression and hostility, a device for gaining attention and sympathy, and an excuse for failure. Tests to determine personality characteristics unique to people who stutter suffer from problems of validity and reliability.

5. **Conditioning theories:** These include the approach-avoidance conflict (Sheehan, 1958) and operant conditioning (Goldiamond, 1965; Shames & Sherrick, 1963). Researchers who based their theories on the operant conditioning paradigm

($S^D{\rightarrow}R{\rightarrow}S^r$) have focused on the performance (R) and the consequent event (S^r), but, as noted above, have not been present at the events that set the occasion for the initial occurrence of the performance.

A hypothesis of the moment of stuttering that was popular at the time Wendell Johnson was conducting research at the University of Iowa was *anticipatory avoidance*. It was refined later by Bloodstein (more recently in 1997) as anticipatory struggle. Bloodstein, as Johnson before him, contends that stuttering is not an organic or a neurotic disorder. Rather, it results from speech specific doubts, which cause the person who stutters to do things that interfere with the motor performance that is intrinsic to speech. He defines stuttering as a sociomotor disorder. The speaker's doubts, his belief that speech is difficult, lead to responses that disrupt the skilled motor performance that is speech. As noted below, doubt is not synonymous with anxiety, nor does it lead to anxiety. People who stutter tense the speech-related muscles and break up or fragment the speech attempt. Stuttering is what speakers do; it is not something that happens to them. Stuttering is not involuntary. It is a consequence of the speaker's actions, and these actions interfere with the motor planning necessary for fluent speech performance.

Even though stuttering represents anticipatory struggle behavior, it is not a function of anxiety about speech or about stuttering. Stuttering is not the anxiety-motivated avoidance of normal disfluencies. Bloodstein rejects anxiety as being basic to stuttering because fluency failures occur even when physiologic arousal, expressed concern, and avoidance responses are absent. Stuttering has not been greatly or consistently reduced by tranquilizers, desensitization, or various forms of psychotherapy. Therefore, anxiety is not a necessary condition for the occurrence of stuttering.

A history of speech failures and the presence of doubt are necessary but not sufficient to cause stuttering. Speech pressure is also a necessary condition, and it may have any number of sources, such as cultural, social, and/or parental attitudes and practices that stress the importance of speech and the need to meet stringent standards. The speech-related pressure combines, in a destructive way, with the doubts that speech failures create.

These doubts and pressures are present in the world of all children, not only for those who are labeled as stuttering. All children exhibit disfluencies and some degree of tension and fragmentation. They all tend to evidence some part-word repetitions and prolongations, disfluent behaviors generally seen as characteristic of stuttering.

What came to be known as Iowa therapy rejected the focus of speech therapy on making an individual stop stuttering. It was thought that stuttering was the effort to avoid stuttering. Therefore, Iowa therapy, as reflected in the work of Bryngelson, Johnson, and Van Riper, among others, essentially instructed the disfluent individual to go ahead and stutter, but to do so in a way that was less likely to result in struggle and avoidant behavior.

A major focus of theories of the moment of stuttering has been on the words or the sounds on which an individual stuttered. Some of these ideas may not be supported by data, even in seemingly obvious instances. For example, Bloodstein, in his retirement address at the CUNY Graduate Center, noted that a disfluent individual who says "b-b-b-baby" will report that he cannot say the /b/ sound. The problem is rather, according to Bloodstein, that the individual who stutters says /b/ exceptionally well, when repeating or prolonging it. The difficulty is with words beginning with /b/. The present author has noted a similar phenomenon among adults with nonfluent (Broca's) aphasia, who stuttered premorbidly. As the fluency impairment from aphasia improved, with an increased ability to produce substantive words in sequence, the individual's stuttering was revealed.

Linguistic Properties of Stuttering

Each individual stutters in a characteristic way. There are no linguistic universals and few observations about individuals who stutter and stuttering that qualify as facts.

Phonologic Properties

Initial sounds of words are affected. Repetitions are more likely to be "re-re-repeat," than "repeat-peat-peat," and prolongations more likely to be "rrrun," than "runnn". There is a *consonant-*

vowel distinction where, on average, there is more stuttering on consonants than on vowels. However, for some people who stutter, a majority of their fluency failures are on vowels. The consonant-vowel distinction is not as strong as the initial sound property. No particular set of consonants is consistently associated with stuttering in a majority of individuals, but a person may typically stutter on certain consonants or class of consonants, such as fricatives or stops. The claim that true stuttering includes the schwa vowel, but normal disfluency does not (e.g., "buh-buh-baby" and "bay-bay-baby," respectively) is probably an oversold notion. In fact, part-word repetitions tend to be produced with vowels that are reduced in stress, and all vowels, when unstressed, tend to migrate toward the schwa.

Morphologic Properties

"Morphologic" is used to describe factors relating to the structure of individual words. Most people who stutter feel that some words are more difficult than others, with word length and frequency of occurrence appearing as significant variables. Regarding *length*, longer words tend to be stuttered more frequently than shorter words in oral reading as well as in conversational speech. Three hypotheses that consider this phenomenon are: they require a greater number of articulatory gestures; they convey more meaning (but see below); and they require more rapid coarticulation than do shorter words. Length of tone unit has been shown to be positively related to stuttering frequency (Howell, Au-Yeung, & Pilgrim, 1999). In terms of *word frequency*, words used less frequently are stuttered more often than those that are used more frequently. However other factors, such as length (longer words are used less frequently) and grammatic class (to be discussed next) confound the study of stuttering with regard to linguistic variables.

Grammatic Properties

Position of a word in a given sentence is a robust factor. The first three words tend to be stuttered more often than subsequent words. Probability of stuttering is highest for the first word of a sentence and lowest for the very last word. This position effect is much more consistent in oral reading than in conversational speech. Also, words at the beginning of a grammatic clause are more likely to be stuttered, particularly for children, than those at the end of clauses. However, this hypothesis has not been tested with right-branching, left-branching, and center-embedded clauses to determine position effect. It may be possible to measure disfluencies in oral reading of such clauses as "to catch the train" in three contexts, randomizing order of presentation: L-branching: *To catch the train*, the man ran up the stairs. C-embedded: The man, *to catch the train*, ran up the stairs. R-branching: The man ran up the stairs *to catch the train*. In terms of *grammatic class*, content words (e.g., adjectives, nouns, adverbs, verbs) elicit more and function words (e.g., pronouns, conjunctions, prepositions, articles) elicit fewer disfluencies for adults. However, very young children who stutter tend to be more disfluent on function words, especially pronouns and conjunctions, than on content words. Linguistic stress relates to increased stuttering in adolescents and adults, and to some degree, in children (Natke, Sandrieser, van Ark, Pietrowsky, & Kalveram, 2004). Speech samples of 22 preschool children indicated that there were significant differences in first-syllable stuttering frequency of function words with short stressed and intermediately stressed syllables than on unstressed syllables.

The presumption that content words are associated with more stuttering and function words with less stuttering for adults is an example of the difficulty inherent in a language analysis of stuttering. These findings may be more apparent than real. Content words are more likely to start with consonants than with vowels; the opposite is true for function words. There are also more function words found in the initial position of sentences and clauses.

An exchange of Letters to the Editor of the *Journal of Speech, Language, and Hearing Research* reveals the intensity of opinion regarding the content versus function word dichotomy. Whole-word repetitions tend to characterize disfluencies on function words, a phenomenon which Wingate (2003) suggests may be indicative of normal disfluency, rather than stuttering, in young children. According to a "generalized adaptation hypothesis"

(Dayalu, Kalinowski, & Stuart, 2003; Dayalu, Kalinowski, Stuart, Holbert, & Rastatter, 2002), repetition of a limited number of function words in meaningful speech results in greater fluency for function than content words. Wingate (2003) also noted that assessment of stuttering via word lists instead of connected speech colors the results of the research, while Dayalu et al. suggest that "the use of word lists is the only scientific method to account and control" for generalized adaptation (2003, p. 1472).

Regarding *grammatic complexity*, there is increased stuttering on sentences that are grammatically more complex. Thus, there is increased stuttering on negative sentences and on sentences that involve the passive form. An experiment to test this hypothesis might control various transformations from the simple, active, affirmative, declarative form. Do two transformations increase stuttering more than one? How much more?

Communicative Properties

It is well known that people who stutter typically exhibit more stuttering in some situations than in others. For example, they may be fluent when talking with small children, close friends, pets, and themselves; very disfluent when talking to a group of people, bosses, or persons in any kind of authority. There may be increased stuttering in situations associated with a high degree of communicative responsibility and propositional (meaningful) speech. The Demands and Capacities (DC) model (Starkweather, 1987; Starkweather, Gottwald, & Halfond, 1990) addresses communicative demand. The premise of the DC model is that "fluency breaks down when environmental and/or self-imposed demands exceed the speaker's cognitive, environmental, and/or emotional capacities for responding" (Adams, 1990, pp. 136–137).

Semantic Properties

Meaningfulness has been examined in oral reading, where there was no difference in the frequency of disfluencies evoked by meaningful and meaningless passages. The increase in stuttering on words with a high information load may be related to semantic factors. However, alternative explanations are that stuttering increases because these words are longer and are used less frequently in communication.

In summary, it is clear that there are many linguistic aspects of stuttering, and many more aspects that are inconsistent, contradictory, unsupported, and untested. Adults who stutter demonstrate lexical and syntactic abilities in comprehension and production similar to fluent peers. However, electrophysiologic testing of linguistic variables in individuals who stutter, using event-related brain potentials, suggests differences in functional brain organization (Weber-Fox, 2001). One observation about linguistic properties is the similarity in descriptions of stuttering to those of apraxia of speech. In the definition below, the word "stuttering" appears in brackets every time the phrase "apraxia of speech" is cited. The result is a pretty serviceable description of the linguistic characterics of both disorders. Similar to stuttering, the term "apraxia of speech" is subject to varying interpretation (Martin, 1974), with the Boston school considering it to be a language disorder associated with Broca's aphasia, and an alternative consideration of apraxia of speech as an articulation disorder, according to the Mayo Clinic school of thought. The definition below is consistent with the latter interpretation.

Apraxia of speech (stuttering) is an articulation disorder that is not accompanied by significant weakness, slowness, or incoordination; muscles involved can be used in reflex and automatic acts. It results from impairment of the capacity to order the positioning of speech musculature and the sequencing of muscle movements for volitional production of phonemes and sequences of phonemes. Symptoms of apraxia of speech (stuttering) include the following: numerous phonemic errors, phonemic error inconsistency, difficulty with initiation of speech, increasing number of phonemic errors with increasing word length, discrepancy between speech perception that may be good and speech production that may be poor, and increased number of errors in oral reading on nouns, verbs, adjectives, and adverbs because they carry linguistic or psychologic weight (Darley, 1964).

Neurophysiologic Properties of Stuttering

For nearly 20 years, Anne Smith has received major funding from the National Institute of Deafness and Other Communication Disorders (R01-DC000559) to study physiologic correlates of stuttering. Her work proceeds from a hypothesis that the etiology of stuttering is the child's failure to acquire stable motor control and coordination for speech, lagging behind normally fluent peers. Decreased speech motor stability has also been reported in adults who stutter as a function of linguistic demands to produce a more complex utterance (Kleinow & Smith, 2000). Bloodstein's (1995) exhaustive description of the physical constitution of the person who stutters organizes the literature in terms of either physiologic processes or lateral dominance. The first group includes breathing movements, where there was no evidence of abnormal diaphragmatic movements during silent breathing; no differences in heart rate, blood pressure, or basal metabolism rate; and no differences in chemical composition of the blood. Where differences were observed in stuttering, as in bilateral dissimilarities of action potentials in musculature such as the masseter, or in observations of tremors, it was not possible to determine if they were a cause or an effect of stuttering. In summary, results do not demonstrate conclusively that the average person who stutters exhibits any clinical pathology in the above factors. The factors observed may have resulted from the influence of excitement, emotion, muscular effort, or fatigue.

Lateral dominance theories were characterized by observations of handedness and reversal of manual dexterity. Early studies found various proportions of stuttering (from 2%–17%) as a result of interference with handedness. These studies did not consider the early onset of stuttering, which is pre-school for most individuals. In fact 80% of people who stuttered and who had shifted handedness had begun to stutter before receiving any instruction in writing. In surveys of hand usage or preference, it was realized that handedness was not an all-or-nothing property, such as maleness, but a matter of degree. There may be some activities where the reader will show preferences for the nondominant hand. Try these tasks as well: fold your hands, and see which thumb is on top; fold your arms, and see which hand is above the elbow. There is no dextrality quotient. People who stutter are relatively right-handed, as are most other people.

Finally, cerebral dominance was measured for language and speech. In the Wada test, sodium amytal is injected into the left carotid artery (which distributes to the zone of language through the middle cerebral artery). If the patient temporarily loses the ability to speak, it is clear that the patient has left-hemisphere dominance for language. By injecting each artery it is determined on which side dominance lies (or if language is represented in both hemispheres). Results of studies indicated that stuttering did not seem to have much to do with impaired cerebral dominance for language; brain injury possibly did.

Persons who stutter have been queried, cajoled, and cut, probed, poked, and punctured, motivated by a science that has not yet explained either the etiology or the moment of stuttering. Johnson's diagnosogenic/semantogenic theory of the onset of stuttering is considered the first well-reasoned theory of stuttering etiology (Wall & Myers, 1995). It would appear that there has been inadequate progress since that early time. The frustration expressed in Perkins' (1997) account of the state of stuttering theory is almost audible. His description (p. 218) of the "hodge-podge" includes the following:

A theory of onset;

A different theory of normal disfluency;

Several theories of how normal disfluency becomes abnormal stuttering;

A theory of primary stuttering and another theory of secondary stuttering;

Separate theories of neurogenic stuttering, developmental stuttering, linguistic stuttering, and articulatory stuttering;

A theory of genetic stuttering;

A theory of cluttering stuttering;

to name a few.

Schuell, Jenkins, and Jimenez-Pabon (1964) noted that what you do about aphasia depends on what you think aphasia is. Although there is legitimate debate about loss versus reduction of efficiency of language comprehension and production, there is nearly universal agreement that damage to specific brain centers generally underlie the deficits. There is no such consensus regarding the etiology or the moment of stuttering. This chapter concludes with an attempt to raise the consciousness of those who would undertake research, especially in an atheoretical discipline.

Power of Professor

Power of attorney has been part of General Business Law since 1948 (Schlesinger, 1990; 1991; Schlesinger & Lavner, 1995). General power of attorney includes durable and nondurable forms, with the former continuing in effect even if the individual who grants the power becomes disabled or incompetent. Power of attorney does not authorize anyone to make medical or other health care decisions, which require a separate health care proxy. When one or more individuals sign(s) a document with power of attorney, the signature must be followed by the phrase "attorney-in-fact" (as opposed to "attorney-at-law").

Power of attorney relates to real estate transactions; chattel and goods transactions; bond, share and commodity transactions; banking transactions; business operating transactions; insurance transactions; estate transactions; claims and litigation; personal relationships and affairs; benefits from military service; records, reports and statements; retirement benefit transactions; making gifts to one's spouse, children and more remote descendants, and parents, not to exceed in the aggregate $10,000 to each of such persons in any year; tax matters; all other matters; and full and unqualified authority to the attorney(s)-in-fact to delegate any or all of the foregoing powers to any person or persons whom the attorney(s)-in-fact shall select.

Nondurable general power of attorney gives a designated person powers to handle property, acting as an agent. These powers end if the person designating the power becomes disabled or incompetent. The powers permits the assigned individual to mortgage, sell, or dispose of any real or personal property without advance notice or approval. This power does not authorize anyone to make medical or other health care decisions, which require a health care proxy.

There have been many historical and statutory notes that expand, limit, qualify, and clarify the powers of attorney, but which have not changed them in substantive ways.

Just as the above powers are consistent with the duties of a licensed attorney-at-law, the power to conduct research is consistent with the duties of a professor. The job description of any university professor is likely to include references to the three areas of academic instruction; service to department, school, university, and professional organizations; and research, including publication in refereed, peer-reviewed journals. The proposal here is to begin a discussion of what constitutes power of professor and what obligations an individual, professor or not, has before being permitted to do research. Following are some preliminary thoughts.

The bulk of the following discussion relates to the "doing" of research, considering the welfare and confidentiality of patients and participants. There is also the major issue of the need for theory. Preparation for power of professor should also include an understanding of types of research, threats to reliability and validity (internal and external), philosophy of science, and the relationships among theory, research, and therapy. It is useful to study the history of communication sciences and disorders (see, for example, Goldfarb, 1985) as a field that borrowed from medicine in Europe (where Emil Froeschels was chief physician and speech pathologist at the University of Vienna in 1918) and from psychology, speech, physics, psychiatry, neurology, and otolaryngology in the United States (the curriculum undertaken by Lee Edward Travis at the University of Iowa in the 1920s for the first Ph.D.-level training in speech and hearing disorders). It is also important to know why the masters degree (and increasingly, the doctorate) is minimal education for safe practice; why speech-language pathology, unlike occupational and physical therapies, is not a prescribed practice; and how reflective clinicianship combines the art and science of communication disorders research and management.

Future theoreticians and researchers should also demonstrate understanding of the following topics.

NIH Training Course

Anyone submitting a grant proposal to the National Institutes of Health after 2000 has been required to complete a computer-based training course on the protection of human research subjects. Available (subject to change) at http://ohsr.od.nih.gov, it takes about one hour and permits the printing of a certificate of completion. It is an excellent overview of research ethics, and should be completed by anyone contemplating research with human participants. The Belmont Report Historical Archive is available (subject to change) at http://www.hhs.gov/ohrp/bel montArchive.html and includes interviews with participants of the National Commission for the Protection of Human Subjects of Biomedical and Behavioral Research (1974–1978). There is also a 9-minute video, featuring participants of the commission.

Institutional Review Board (IRB) Research Review Form

Before beginning any research project involving human participants, an investigator must obtain IRB approval. Forms, which are reasonably standard across institutions, generally require a brief description of the project's purposes, methodology, and design; dates for initiation and completion of the project; number and characteristics of participants; method of recruitment; and any potential risks, stresses, or discomforts, and the precautions taken to minimize them. Investigators must include an informed consent form and a representative sample of materials. There may also be a required debriefing form, as well as a sign-up sheet or advertisement.

Health Insurance Portability and Accountability Act of 1996 (HIPAA)

Established by the 104th Congress on August 21, 1996 as Public Law 104-191, HIPAA amended the Internal Revenue Code of 1986, in part to combat waste, fraud, and abuse in health care delivery. The purpose of HIPAA was to establish standards and requirements for electronic transmission of health information and to encourage the development of a health information system. Many aspects of HIPAA are relevant to practitioners in communication sciences and disorders. The term "health information" includes oral or recorded forms, created by a health care provider (such as a speech-language pathologist or audiologist), a school, or a university, which refer to physical or mental health of an individual in the past, present, or future.

Individually identifiable health information is protected. This includes demographic or other physical or mental health information which can reasonably be believed to identify an individual. Security standards and safeguards are incorporated in the 16-page document, as are monetary and incarceration penalties for failure to comply with requirements and standards.

Professional Code of Ethics

The ASHA Board of Ethics began revising the *Code of Ethics* in August 2000, with a focus on ethics in research and professional practice. The Board passed a final version of the proposed revisions in August 2002 and submitted the changes to the Legislative Council, which passed the resolution in November 2002 at the ASHA Convention. The revised *Code of Ethics* took effect in January 2003. Before being revised, the code contained four specific references to research and only two areas: rights and welfare of participants in research, and public statements about research results.

The revisions in Principle of Ethics I add humane treatment of animals to the section on welfare of participants and also address issues of nondiscrimination, informed consent, confidentiality, and security of research data. Principle of Ethics II refers to professional competency. In this section, ASHA incorporates a philosophy similar to that used by physicians in hospitals, where doctors may have general, specialized, or research privileges (Goldfarb, 1989). Research privileges include all general privileges and responsibilities. In addition, some specialized privileges, such as the use of sophisticated instrumentation, may be essential to the implementation of research. Clinical investigators may collaborate with other behavioral scientists and physicians who have research privileges. Finally, Principle of Ethics III requires accurate and honest information about an individual's contributions to research activities.

Research 101

A new generation of scholars in research is needed about every 10 years. The dearth of doctoral-level members of ASHA, particularly among the newer generations, is alarming. In the year the Symposium on Ethics and the Tudor Study was held at the

CUNY Graduate Center, the 13 Ph.D. degrees awarded in speech and hearing sciences at that institution was the most of any university in the nation. It was also a far larger number than subsequent graduating classes, in a doctoral-only institution with 4,000 Ph.D. students.

Research in communication sciences and disorders, which fewer ASHA members will be qualified (by virtue of limited education) to undertake, will still be done. However, if speech and hearing science research is completed by psychologists, linguists, and physicians, then communication sciences and disorders as a separate discipline will lose its legitimacy, perhaps even its right to exist.

With power of professor, an individual with an M.A., M.S., or Au.D. could earn research privileges based on competencies. ASHA might extend the Knowledge and Skills Assessment protocol to research, or a Special Interest Division established to grant power of professor. The energy of this newly empowered generation might serve to make the title of the present chapter obsolete.

References

Adams, M. R. 1990. The demands and capacities model: I. Theoretical elaborations. *Journal of Fluency Disorders, 15*, 135–141.

Ambrose, N. G., Cox, N. J., & Yairi, E. (1997). The genetic basis of persistence and recovery in stuttering. *Journal of Speech, Language, and Hearing Research, 40*, 567–580.

Anderson, B. (1971). *The psychology experiment.* Belmont, CA: Brooks/ Cole.

Bloodstein, O. (1995). *A handbook on stuttering.* San Diego, CA: Singular Publishing Group.

Bloodstein, O. (1997). Stuttering as an anticipatory struggle reaction. In R. F. Curlee & G. M. Siegel (Eds.), *Nature and treatment of stuttering* (2nd ed., pp. 169–181) Boston: Allyn & Bacon.

Darley, F. L. (1964). *Diagnosis and appraisal of communicative disorders.* Englewood Cliffs, NJ: Prentice-Hall.

Dayalu, V. N., Kalinowski, J., & Stuart, A. (2003). Interpreting differences in stuttering frequency on content and function words: A reply to Wingate (2003). *Journal of Speech, Language, and Hearing Research, 46*, 1471–1472.

Dayalu, V. N., Kalinowski, J., Stuart, A., Holbert, D., & Rastatter, M. P. (2002). Stuttering frequency on content and function words in adults who stutter: A concept revisited. *Journal of Speech, Language, and Hearing Research, 45,* 871–878.

Freeman, F., & Ushijima, T. (1978). Laryngeal muscle activity during stuttering. *Journal of Speech and Hearing Research, 21,* 538–562.

Goldfarb, R. (1985). Speech handicaps/communication disorders. In T. Husen & T. N. Postlethwaite (Eds.), *International encyclopedia of education* (pp. 4760–4766). Oxford: Pergamon.

Goldfarb, R. (1989). Organization of speech, language, and hearing programmes in United States hospitals. *The College of Speech Therapists Bulletin, 452,* 2–7.

Goldiamond, I. (1965). Stuttering and fluency as manipulatable operant response classes. In L. Krasner, & L. P. Ullmann (Eds.), *Research in behavior modification.* New York: Holt, Rinehart & Winston.

Hawking, S. (2001). *The universe in a nutshell.* New York: Bantam.

Howell, P., Au-Yeung, J., & Pilgrim, L. (1999). Utterance rate and linguistic properties as determinants of lexical dysfluencies in children who stutter. *Journal of the Acoustical Society of America, 105,* 481–490.

Kleinow, J., & Smith, A. (2000). Influences of length and syntactic complexity on the speech motor stability of the fluent speech of adults who stutter. *Journal of Speech, Language, and Hearing Research, 43,* 548–559.

Kuhn, T. W. (1962). *The structure of scientific revolutions.* Chicago: University of Chicago Press.

Martin, A., D., 1974. Some objections to the term "apraxia of speech." *Journal of Speech and Hearing Disorders, 39,* 53–64.

Myers, F. (1996). Cluttering: A matter of perspective. *Journal of Fluency Disorders, 21,* 175–185.

Natke, U., Sandrieser, P., van Ark, M., Pietrowsky, R., & Kalveram, K. T. (2004). Linguistic stress, within-word position, and grammatical class in relation to early childhood stuttering. *Journal of Fluency Disorders, 29,* 109–122.

Perkins, W. H. (1997). Stuttering: Why science hasn't solved it. In. R. F. Curlee & G. M. Siegel (Eds.), *Nature and treatment of stuttering* (2nd ed., pp. 218–235). Boston: Allyn & Bacon.

Schiavetti, N., & Metz, D.E. (2002). *Evaluating research in communicative disorders* (4th ed.). Boston: Allyn & Bacon.

Schlesinger, S. J. (1990). Personal planning with powers of attorney. *Brooklyn Barrister, 41,* 178.

Schlesinger, S. J. (1991). "Pros" and "cons" of revocable living trusts (part II). *Brooklyn Barrister, 43,* 19.

Schlesinger, S. J., & Lavner, S. (1995). Statutory short form powers of attorney. *New York State Bar Journal, 67,* 18.

Schuell, H. M., Jenkins, J. J., & Jimenez-Pabon, E. (1964). *Aphasia in adults.* New York: Harper and Row.

Schwartz, M. (1976). *Stuttering solved.* New York: Lippincott.

Shames, G. H., & Sherrick, C. E. (1963). A discussion of nonfluency and stuttering as operant behavior. *Journal of Speech and Hearing Disorders, 28,* 3–18.

Sheehan, J. G. (1958). Conflict theory of stuttering. In J. Eisenson (Ed.), *Stuttering: a symposium* (pp. 121–166). New York: Harper and Row.

Skinner, B. F. (1972). *Cumulative record.* New York: Appleton-Century-Crofts.

Starkweather, C. W., 1987. *Fluency and stuttering.* Englewood Cliffs, NJ: Prentice-Hall.

Starkweather, C. W., Gottwald, S. R., & Halfond, M. M. (1990). *Stuttering prevention: A clinical method.* Englewood Cliffs, NJ: Prentice-Hall.

Wall, M. J., & Myers, F. L. (1995). *Clinical management of childhood stuttering* (2nd ed.). Austin, TX: Pro-Ed.

Watkins, M. (1981). Human memory and the information-processing metaphor. *Cognition, 10,* 331–336.

Weber-Fox, C. (2001). Neural systems for sentence processing in stuttering. *Journal of Speech, Language, and Hearing Research, 44,* 814–825.

West, R., & Nussbaum, E. (1929). A motor test for dysphemia. *Quarterly Journal of Speech, 15,* 469-479.

Wingate, M. (1977). The relationship of theory to therapy in stuttering. *Journal of Communication Disorders, 10,* 37–44.

Wingate, M. E. (2003). Major problems with a revisit. *Journal of Speech, Language, and Hearing Research, 46,* 1468–1470.

Yairi, E. (1997). Home environments and parent-child interaction in childhood stuttering. In R. F. Curlee, & G. M. Siegel (Eds.), *Nature and treatment of stuttering: New directions* (2nd ed., pp. 24–48). Boston: Allyn & Bacon.

Yairi, E., & Ambrose, N. (1992). Onset of stuttering in preschool children: Selected factors. *Journal of Speech and Hearing Research, 35,* 782–788.

Yairi, E., Ambrose, N., & Cox, N. (1996). Genetics of stuttering: A critical review. *Journal of Speech and Hearing Research, 39,* 771–784.

Yairi, E., Ambrose, N., Paden., E., & Throneburg, R. N. (1996). Predictive factors of persistence and recovery: Pathways of childhood stuttering. *Journal of Communication Disorders, 29,* 51–77.

9

RETROACTIVE ETHICAL JUDGMENTS AND HUMAN SUBJECTS RESEARCH

The 1939 Tudor Study in Context[1]

Nicholas Johnson

However significant speech pathology research may be, its publication is seldom the focus of the kind of national media attention that the Tudor study received during the summer of 2001.

That the media's spotlight was focused, not on a new discovery, but on ethical judgments regarding Mary Tudor's then 62-year-old little masters thesis about speech disfluency (Tudor, 1939) should have made university and association administrators, speech pathologists, and journalists a little skeptical as to why this was considered "news." Some were.

Indeed, as will be seen, the ethical issues surrounding the study turn out to involve the ethics of journalism and administration as much or more than the ethics of human subjects research.

The barrage of ethical and moral accusations hurled at the surviving researcher, and her then-36-years-dead supervisor, Dr. Wendell Johnson, were driven by a couple of articles by Jim Dyer in the *San Jose Mercury News* (Dyer, 2001).[2] The articles were treated as a major exposé, widely distributed by the *Mercury News*, and reprinted all across the country.

There is a noteworthy contrast between the 2001 coverage of the 1939 study by the *Mercury News,* and the 2001 coverage of a 2001 study by the *Baltimore Sun* (Siegel & Sugg, 2001). The former study involved no physical contact with subjects, no use of harmful substances, and, the best evidence suggests, no permanent harm. It was conducted by a young masters student with a handful of subjects 62 years earlier. The 2001 study involved subjects' ingestion of harmful substances, produced a possibly predictable *death* of a subject, and occurred at the hands of professional researchers at one of the nation's most prestigious institutions that very year.

The *Mercury News* reporter ignored the more dramatic late 20th century ethical lapses resulting in serious harm to human subjects. He chose instead to cast moral aspersions on what he charged a masters student and her supervisor had done 62 years earlier.

The *Sun's* series of stories, by contrast, skipped the Tudor study and avoided emotion-laden charges. They profiled the Hopkins researcher and provided an explanation both of the need for oversight and the harm that comes from overreaction. They explored the most appropriate public relations stance for an institution in this position and some of the conflict of interest issues that arise when academic research is funded by corporations impacted by the results. In short, by putting the story in context, the *Sun* was able to explore some of the broader issues for its readers and, in this writer's opinion, use its editorial page responsibly.

Why the *Mercury News* reporter was motivated to do what he did remains unknown. What *is* known is that he "resigned" shortly after his stories appeared and his own ethical lapses were revealed (see section VII. D., below).

Sadly, however, the damage had already been done. The advice attributed to Mark Twain, "never pick a fight with someone who buys printer's ink by the barrel," is still applicable. Media damage, once done, can almost never be fully repaired; truth is a notoriously slow runner in its race with defamation.

Responses to the ethical charges leveled at the researcher and her supervisor can be summarized as follows:

1. **If harm was neither intended nor done, that really ought to be the end of the matter.** If some of the critics of the *sub-*

stance of the Tudor study are correct (i.e., that she drew unwarranted conclusions from her data), Tudor not only could not have, and did not, produce "stuttering" in her subjects, neither did she do them any other permanent harm. Moreover, say the critics, there is no evidence that she or her supervisor *intended* to do any permanent harm.

Human subjects researcher Dr. Michael Flaum wrote a response to his local college paper's editorial criticizing Tudor's ethics. After reviewing the evidence he wrote, "That really ought to be the end of the matter. If harm was neither intended nor done, what's the problem? Where's the 'lack of ethics' your editorial headlined?" (Flaum, 2002, p. 8A)

2. **Measured by the standards of its time.** Assume permanent harm *was* done to some subjects, even though the best evidence suggests none occurred. But even were that true, scholarly thoroughness and basic fairness require that Tudor's procedures be judged by the human subjects research standards of 1939 (when the study was done) not those of 2001 (when the criticisms were leveled).

   Indeed, why would anyone even *want* to be morally judgmental (as distinguished from descriptive or analytic)? Why would anyone *want* to judge the research procedures of a 1939 study by the human subjects ethical standards of 2001, 62 years later? That is as inappropriate as it would be to use the ethical standards of 2063 to look back upon our behavior in 2001.

   In any event, as a former university vice president for research has said of the ethics of the Tudor study, "it was fully within the norms of the time" (Dyer, 2001).[3]

3. **Measured by today's standards.** Now make *two* false assumptions: that harm *was* done, *and* that the most appropriate baseline for evaluating the Tudor study's ethics are the human subjects standards of 2001. At a minimum, the procedures used by Tudor compare very favorably with those used by some researchers in prestigious U.S. institutions since 1939, even some since 1995.

4. **Indictment or itemization?** Given the abuses in post-World War II human subjects research, if one is interested in

exploring and improving the ethical standards applicable to twenty-first century research the Tudor study seems a trivial, dated, and unproductive example to choose.

If one wishes to examine it anyway, the only responsible approach is to itemize the qualities and procedures of that study one at a time. What *specifically* is it about the Tudor study that is thought to be unethical? When the analysis is approached in that way there are few, if any, aspects of the study one can fairly criticize.

5. **Administrative ethics.** Responses to the Tudor study provide insights not only into journalistic ethics, and human subjects research ethics, but administrative ethics as well.

Following the *Mercury News* stories, the reaction by some university and association administrators and speech pathologists was a prompt and forceful indictment of the ethics of the researcher and her supervisor. This response bore a stark contrast to their response, and that of their predecessors, to the publicity involving harm to human subjects for which *they* bore some responsibility. From the post-World War II abuses through the post-1995 scandals, human subjects research abuses often provoked no response whatsoever from responsible administrators—until those abuses were publicized. Even then, all too often, the response of administrators and researchers in industry, research institutions and the academy was one of defensiveness rather than apologies and calls for reform.[4]

Such responses understandably leave the impression, whether fairly or not, that researchers' and administrators' primary concern may be public relations and continued funding. The welfare of their human subjects and the harm done to them seldom produce even comment, let alone action.

Given this history, one can only speculate as to why administrators were so quick to chastise Tudor. Perhaps it was their confidence that ethical rectitude regarding 62-year-old studies could only enhance, rather than threaten, their research budgets.

6. **Scholarship, scandals, and the ethics of ethical criticism.** An evaluation of the *substance* of the Tudor study—the adequacy of its design, reliability of the data, and soundness of

the conclusions—is beyond the scope of this chapter. It is the subject of other chapters. But the writer shares the view that if the Tudor study's data are subject to a more accurate analysis today than when first gathered, that analysis should be done, reported, and published, as it has been (Ambrose & Yairi, 2002).

Similarly, the ethical issues surrounding the study also can be explored in a dispassionate, analytical, and scholarly way.

The writer's primary objection relates to those criticisms of the study's ethics that have been as full of emotionalism as they have been empty of factual analysis and serious reflection, such as the headlined characterization of it as "the monster study."[5] Such criticisms are similar to the thought-less repetition of harmful, inaccurate, and uncorroborated gossip that sometimes creates legal liability for defamation. There *should be*, in short, an ethics of ethical criticism.

7. **Journalist, Heal Thyself.** Finally, and central to the chapter, is journalistic ethics.

In 1939 the research community had not yet written and agreed to the international human subjects research standards that would only come decades later. The University of Iowa had in place neither standards nor a process for reviewing their compliance. Thus, none could have been violated. Moreover, the Tudor study complied with most of those that have evolved since. The best evidence is that no permanent harm appears to have been done to any of Tudor's subjects.

By contrast, there *were* applicable journalistic ethical standards in 2001. They *were* violated. And those violations *have* caused harm (see section VII. D., below).

I. Neither Harm nor Intention to Harm

Nicoline Grinager Ambrose and Ehud Yairi are critical of the conclusions that Mary Tudor drew from her data. When they reanalyzed her original data they concluded there were no sig-nificant changes in disfluency of *any* type in *any* of the four groups tested. As is fully explained elsewhere in this book, there was certainly no direct evidence of "stuttering" based on changes in the speech of participants.[6]

Given that they are severe critics of the study and not its apologists, it is the more credible and commendable that they are able to bring such scholarly balance and dispassion to their analysis of Tudor's ethics. They report their belief that no harm was done to the subjects, in the sense of "instilling chronic stuttering," and that there was no intention to do harm.[7]

II. Compared to What?

A. What Is Human Subjects Research?

"Human subjects research," as the phrase suggests, is research for which the laboratory test tube and animal studies are inadequate. It must involve humans if it is to be done at all. A common example would be the testing of a new pharmaceutical product. In 2001, before a new drug could be sold to the public the manufacturer had to demonstrate that it would not do serious harm, that it would alleviate whatever condition it is designed to cure, and that its side effects are known and communicated (FDA, 1962).

This process usually requires that the drug be tested on humans during "clinical trials," often conducted by researchers in academic institutions. Those who participate in those trials are called human subjects.

B. The Evolution of Human Subjects Research Ethics

Over time, thinking has shifted regarding the ethical issues raised by human subjects research. The standards of the nineteenth century are different from those in 1939, 2001, and what those standards will evolve to become by 2063. For example, in 2001 there was greater sensitivity regarding the use of prisoners and institutionalized children as subjects than there was during the 19th and early 20th centuries.

Similarly, in the 20th century there was a stark disparity in the ethical standards applied by American researchers to human subjects in North America compared to their subjects in developing countries.[8] This practice, seldom even questioned let alone criticized at the time, may come to be viewed by mid-21st century critics as having been highly unethical.

During the last half of the 20th century, there was much progress in the thinking regarding ethics in human subjects research. Many more regulations and opportunities for review were put in place. It is still possible for harm to occur. It is still probable that future ethicists will look backward, condemning with the standards of their day practices widely accepted in 2001. But either is much less likely than a century, half-century, or even decade before 2001.

The research community can be rightfully proud of that progress. At the same time, two things must be said.

1. Ethical violations causing harm to human subjects will still occur, whether measured by the articulated standards of 2001 or the standards that will evolve.

2. Pendulums have a tendency to swing beyond the midpoint. This may have happened with human subjects research ethical standards. That is, some of the early twenty-first century standards may be inhibiting needed research while producing little benefit.[9]

C. The Four Phases of Ethical Evolution

In evaluating the evolution of human subjects research ethics it is useful to identify, albeit somewhat arbitrarily, four phases of ethical evolution.

Phase I includes roughly the 19th and first half of the 20th centuries. During this phase, there were "ethics" in general, and even occasional comments about human subjects research in particular, but few if any officially promulgated and universally agreed-on human subjects research standards. The ethical standards, like the research designs, were left almost entirely to individual researchers.

Phase II, the primary focus of this historical section of the chapter, is the period from World War II through the 1970s. This is the time when abuses came to public attention, consciousness was raised, and international ethical standards evolved, were drafted, adopted, and published.

Phase III is the 1980s and 1990s, when new standards were finally in place and applied.

Phase IV is the last five years of the 20th century, a period when concerns and procedures were at their most intricate, intense, and some would say self-defeating stage so far (e.g., Shea, 2000).

Phases I, III, and IV are dealt with only in passing. The illustrations selected from Phase II, described below, will be referred to throughout the remainder of the chapter.

D. From World War II Through the 1970s[10]

Following World War II a review of experiments conducted by German researchers resulted in what came to be called the Nuremberg Code of 1948.[11] It provided that human subjects research should involve only subjects who give informed consent and volunteer to participate.

The code is significant because it marks the beginning of Phase II. The first time such standards were ever set forth in an international agreement was 1948, nine years *after* the 1939 Tudor study. This was followed by the World Medical Association's Declaration of Helsinki, adopted a quarter century after Tudor, and most recently revised in 2000.[12] It spells out some additional requirements, such as the suggestion that laboratory and animal research should precede human subjects research.

It is worth noting, however, that even these most rigorous standards do not forbid the taking of risks in human subjects research. The necessary finding is simply that "risks to subjects are reasonable relative to anticipated benefits . . . and the importance of the knowledge that may reasonably be expected to result."[13]

The reader should also bear in mind that none of the experiments described below were done by a lone researcher in a secret laboratory outside the control of reputable research institutions and other controls. These are studies done by well-educated, accomplished, and respected professionals. Most were reviewed and funded by additional professionals and institutions. They were often published in peer-reviewed academic journals. Few or no questions of their propriety appear to have been raised about them by anyone at any stage.

Note also that, unlike the 1939 Tudor study, all were done *after* ethical standards and regulations were in place, standards that would seem to have been violated by one or more aspects of the studies.

1. The Tuskegee Syphilis Study

One of the most often-cited illustrations of the ethical problems in human subjects research is the Tuskegee syphilis study. Like other human subjects research studies of the time, it was designed and conducted by highly educated, professional physicians, in this instance those with the U.S. Public Health Service (PHS).

Over 400 African-Americans with syphilis were recruited. Not only did the subjects not provide informed consent to their participation, they were affirmatively *misinformed* that they would receive "special free treatment." They were not informed of the nature of their disease or that the research would offer them no therapeutic benefit.

Their complications got worse. Their death rate became twice that of the control subjects. Yet the study continued. Even after penicillin became available, and was known to be effective in the treatment of syphilis, the men were neither informed of this nor treated. When outside doctors diagnosed a subject as having the disease researchers intervened to *prevent* treatment.

In 2001, research professionals and even many members of the public were aware of this study. What was not so widely known was that the Tuskegee study *continued from 1932 until 1973*, long after the Nuremberg Code and Helsinki Declaration were in existence and well known.

How could this be? Was it because the study continued for too brief a time, or was unknown to the research community? No, it continued over a period of 40 years and was widely reported in medical journals.

One of today's administrative protections of subjects' rights is the oversight of human subjects research by an institutional review board, or IRB. A researcher's colleagues must review and approve each study and find that it complies with current administrative regulations, institutional procedures, and ethical standards.

Were there no IRBs at that time? No, that cannot be the answer either. Earlier versions of an IRB were in place. The

Tuskegee study was periodically reviewed and approved by Public Health Service officials and medical societies. As a federally funded agency, there may have been Congressional oversight as well.

Today, such agencies and institutions would have detailed regulations in place. Were there no regulations at the PHS at that time? No, that can't be it. The *Public Health Service Policy for the Protection of Human Subjects* became effective six or more years before the study was stopped.

Can one say that the Tuskegee study is merely one unfortunate aberration in an otherwise stellar history of ethical sensitivity and compliance by research institutions? No, unfortunately, the following studies suggest that's not the answer either.

2. Radiation at the "Science Club"

From 1946 to 1956 19 boys who thought they were part of a "science club" were, without their consent or knowledge, drinking radioactive milk provided them by researchers from Harvard and MIT.

3. Calculated Risks from Atomic Bomb Testing

Radiated milk is one thing. But in 1949 the Atomic Energy Commission wanted to know whether the fallout from its atomic bomb tests could threaten the viability of all life on earth. Apparently, knowing the seriousness of the risk, the agency thought it one worth taking. The tests continued, including those it conceded posed a "calculated risk" of radiation exposure to populations living downwind from the tests.

4. Doctors' Patients as Human Research Subjects

Until the 1960s, pharmaceutical companies paid doctors willing to use uninformed patients for human subjects research. Participating doctors were provided free samples by the drug companies, required to keep records of patients' reactions, and then provide those results to the companies. The acceptance of the practice was so widespread that few thought it worthy of comment.

In the 1960s there was no law that required drugs be tested before marketing. Companies did not have to show their products were even safe, let alone useful for the conditions for which they were prescribed.

At that point in the history of human subjects research ethics, America was an entire nation of uninformed, nonconsenting human subjects. The profits from the system went to the pharmaceutical companies and doctors. The losses were borne by their human subjects in the form of occasional injury, disease, and even death.

By 2001, the testing took the form of what were called "clinical trials," often in academic medical centers. Most subjects provided some form of informed consent, thereby relieving the institutions of potential legal liability. But the medicines were still free, the doctors were still compensated by the pharmaceutical companies in a variety of ways, and the health and financial risks still fell upon the subjects.

For example, in August 2001 it was reported that some 81 persons using cholesterol-lowering drugs had died from muscle cell degeneration. Hilts reported that doctors often ignored warnings regarding usage and side effects. As few as 5% of the participating doctors were found to be conducting the essential monthly liver tests of their patients (Hilts, 2001).

5. The Thalidomide Babies

One of the human subjects tests of pharmaceuticals in the 1950s involved a sedative from Germany called thalidomide. It was given to pregnant women to control sleep and nausea. Unfortunately, however useful as a sedative, one of thalidomide's nasty side effects is that it causes missing or deformed limbs and other severe deformities in fetuses. As a result, the human subjects in this research project, almost all of whom were in Europe, gave birth to some 12,000 deformed "thalidomide babies."

These results were so dramatic, widely reported, and accompanied by gruesome photographs, that they led to public and official questioning of the lucrative relationship between doctors and pharmaceutical companies.

6. The Army's Exclusion

In 1962, the U.S. Army addressed human subjects research ethical issues with regard to its experiments on soldiers and others.

The Army wanted data regarding the human impact of weapons of mass destruction (agents used in atomic, chemical, and biological warfare). But with the urging of nonmilitary consultants it expressly *excluded* from its ethical standards "clinical research" involving military personnel.

By 2002, the Defense Department released more than two dozen reports of previously classified exercises from 1962 through 1973. These exercises involved the deliberate exposure of U.S. troops to agents in chemical and biological weapons without the consent, or even knowledge, of the subjects. The agents, "some of the most poisonous in the arsenal," included VX, sarin, soman, tabun, and *Bacillus globigii* (related to anthrax). As of 2002, the Department was trying to track down some 5,500 known subjects (*New York Times*, October 10, 2002).

7. Injecting Cancer

As late as 1963, doctors in a New York hospital were deliberately injecting live cancer cells into subjects. The chief investigator was a physician from the Sloan-Kettering Cancer Research Institute. The study was reviewed and approved by the hospital's medical director. There was no documentation of the subjects' consent, nor were they informed what was being done to them.

Following the disclosure of the study and its procedures there were no immediate repercussions for the hospital, Sloan-Kettering, the university involved, or the U.S. Public Health Service.

8. The Chimpanzee's Kidney Experiment

The same year (1963), a Tulane University doctor performed an unsuccessful transplant of a kidney from a chimpanzee into a human being. The procedure promised no benefit to the recipient or new scientific knowledge. It was funded by the National Institutes of Health after repeated approval as the proposal passed through various levels of review.

9. Giving Hepatitis to the Mentally Retarded

From 1956 to 1972, a New York University doctor led a hepatitis study team at the Willowbrook State School for the Retarded in

New York. The subjects, all of whom were children, were fed extracts of stools from individuals infected with hepatitis.

Did their parents consent? In theory, yes, because there was a "consent form." In reality, no, because the form seemed to suggest that the children were going to receive a vaccine to *protect against* the virus rather than be *deliberately infected*. Moreover, Willowbrook administrators told parents it was overcrowded and unable to take more residents. More precisely, children would not be admitted *unless the parents would first consent* to their children becoming a part of the study, in which case there was plenty of room.

Note that the study very likely could have been done with children who already had the disease, rather than infecting those who did not. Once again, this was not an example of the research of an unsupervised loner. The study was reviewed, approved and funded by the Armed Forces Epidemiological Board. It was further reviewed and approved by the executive faculty of the NYU School of Medicine.

10. NASA's Exception

It was 1968 before NASA came up with an informed consent policy. However, even then the policy provided that the requirement could be waived in a number of circumstances, including when the research *"would be seriously hampered"* if consent had to be obtained.

11. LSD from the CIA

It was not until *1975* that Congressional hearings brought to public attention some of the more questionable human subjects research projects of the CIA and Defense Department. The agencies wanted to know the extent to which it was possible to control human behavior through the use of radiation, psychologic means, psychoactive drugs, such as LSD and mescaline, and other chemical and biological substances. The subjects used in these experiments had not given informed consent, and some died.

The secret project's code name was MKULTRA. It involved at least 150 individually reviewed, approved, and funded projects conducted by presumably reputable research scientists. The CIA director ordered all records of the studies destroyed in 1973.

12. 2005: The Deaths Continue

There is no shortage of such examples—up to and including the present day. To illustrate the point, and conclude this listing, as the book was going to press there were another couple of Associated Press reports of deaths in human subjects research studies. One was a May 5, 2005, story about a then-current NIH study that utilized foster children with AIDS (Associated Press, 2005a). Many of these often poor and minority children were not provided the required child advocates researchers had promised, and some suffered side effects, including increased death rates, as a result of otherwise untested dosages. The story led to a congressional investigation which revealed variations in practices from state-to-state (Associated Press, 2005c). The other was a May 18, 2005, story regarding two deaths and "life-threatening complications in an alarming number of others" resulting from a breast cancer study of the combined effects of two drugs, docetaxel and doxorubicin (Associated Press, 2005b).

III. Administrative Ethics, Complacency, and Opposition to Reform

The relevance of these 12 illustrations are the contrasts between them and the Tudor study in terms of (a) the degree of permanent harm done, (b) the existence of applicable, published ethical standards, (c) the willingness to apply the ethical standards of the day to studies done over half a century earlier, (d) the availability of institutional resources and participation of professionals, and (e) the criticism subsequently leveled at the researcher.

A. The Tuskegee Syphilis Study

What finally stopped the Tuskegee study? It does not appear to have been the ethical concerns of a research community clearly willing to continue for 40 years procedures that violated known ethical standards.

It seems to have been an outraged public that finally prodded Congress into holding hearings on the ethical and legal standards for human subjects research. Even then, *after* all the revelations, Senator Ted Kennedy's bill to create a National Human Experimentation Board, *as recommended by the Tuskegee Syphilis Study Ad Hoc Panel*, was defeated. The hope for oversight of all federally funded research was lost as a result of the efforts of lobbyists for the research community and their corporate sponsors.

Even the compromise, the National Research Act of 1974, was cut back so that the regulations would govern only the Department of Health, Education and Welfare. And those compromised regulations were further watered down, leaving the grantee institutions free to regulate themselves through their self-appointed institutional review boards.

The subsequent *Belmont Report*, spelling out more ethical standards ("respect, beneficence, and justice"), did not appear until 1979 (National Committee for the Protection of Human Subjects, *The Belmont Report*, 1979). The Department of Health and Human Services (DHHS) regulations based on that report became available in 1981. Other governmental agencies did not sign on until 10 years after even that. The DHHS regulations were formally adopted by over a dozen agencies in 1991, 52 years after the Tudor study, and are now referred to as the "Common Rule." And even this set of rules provides for six categories of exemptions.

B. The Thalidomide Babies

The deformities in 12,000 thalidomide babies were one of the most dramatic of human subjects research failures. However, even they were not enough to produce reform. It was only after those deaths had attracted a good deal of *media attention* that Congressional hearings were scheduled and held.

Moreover, notwithstanding the dramatic events, media attention, and hearings, the industry and research community were still able to weaken the legislation. In the end, "informed consent" would be required, but "the best judgment of the doctors involved" would control whether consent was "feasible" or "in the best interests of the patient."

With little or no thanks to the pharmaceutical industry or medical profession, by 2001 the law authorized the Food and Drug Administration (FDA) to insist on the safety and efficacy of new drugs. At that time, the law was still attacked by industry on grounds that it delayed getting drugs to patients. Meanwhile, experiments with thalidomide continue, although hopefully not on pregnant women.

C. Injecting Cancer

As noted above, even after it was revealed that the Sloan-Kettering researchers had been deliberately injecting cancer into human subjects, there were no immediate repercussions for the hospital, Sloan-Kettering, the university involved, or the U.S. Public Health Service. Such professional concern as did exist focused not so much on the ethics of the researchers, and harm to the subjects, as on the possible adverse impact of public knowledge on the continued funding of such research and the possibilities of legal liability.[14]

D. The Chimpanzee's Kidney Experiment

Following revelations of the chimpanzee's kidney experiment, there was a thorough NIH review of "research protocols and procedures." However, the ultimate recommendation was for no changes whatsoever. The agency was concerned that if it promulgated standards they might "inhibit, delay or distort the carrying out of clinical research." One of the nation's primary sources of funding for human subjects research was simply "not in a position to shape the educational foundations of medical ethics."

E. Deaths in Developing Countries

The dual ethical standards applied by American researchers to their human subjects in the U.S. and in developing countries are illustrated by Paul M. McNeill's report (McNeill, 1998). For example, in a Uganda AIDS study, partners of AIDS-infected subjects were not informed and 90 of them (22%) subsequently died.

What was the response of ethical professionals? *AllAfrica Global Media* reported that "The Rakai study was approved by scientific and ethics boards in Uganda and the United States. After the controversy broke out, UNAIDS, the United Nations office that coordinates the international response to the epidemic, found no ethical violations" (AllAfrica Global Media, 2001). For a fictional account of a pharmaceutical company's unethical human subjects research on Africans (said to be based on a true story), see John LeCarré, *The Constant Gardener* (2001). The movie version of the same name, starring Ralph Fiennes and Rachel Weisz, was released and playing in theaters as this book went to press in 2005.

F. The Beecher Report

One person who *did* try to bring attention to some of the earlier questionable studies was a researcher named Henry Beecher. He spoke at a convention of science journalists in 1965. He cited 22 examples of research with potentially serious ethical violations that he had found in published reports in medical journals.

How could this be? Were the authors and editors of these 22 papers unaware of the applicable ethical standards? Aware but uncaring? Or was there some less disturbing explanation? Rather than distance himself from such questions about abuses, Beecher was candid enough to acknowledge that "in years gone by work in my laboratory could have been criticized."

His paper was rejected for publication by the *Journal of the American Medical Association* (JAMA).

IV. Ethical Analysis of the Tudor Study: Indictment or Itemization?

The more one knows of the human subjects research ethical violations described above, and administrators' responses to them *after* standards were in place, the more difficult it becomes to fault the Tudor study. One becomes ever more questioning of why anyone would even think about its ethics 62 years later, let alone make it the poster child for a national media blitz.

Moreover, in doing so, to phrase an ethical inquiry into the Tudor study as a question of "whether it was ethical or unethical" is to reveal one's lack of analysis before the inquiry even begins. The inquiry should not be focused on the study as a whole, but rather on specific aspects of the study's ethics. What *precisely* was it about the study that was or was not ethical? Some of those aspects are listed below. As will be seen, when examined in this way the 1939 Tudor study, conducted at a time when no applicable ethical standards had yet been promulgated, compares very favorably with studies done *after* the existence of those standards.

A. Was There Anything Unethical About the Involvement of Children as Human Subjects?

Although the 2001 standards were quite strict, they still permitted child subjects. Indeed, as Eberlein notes, as many as 95% of children with cancer are today involved in clinical trials (Eberlein, 2000).

Clearly children continued to be a part of many studies during Phase II. Consider, for example, the boys served radioactive milk, the children infected with hepatitis, and the foster children used as subjects in tests of AIDS drugs in 2005.

Because the Tudor study involved a test of a hypothesis about the onset of disfluency in *children*, it was necessary that children be involved if the study was to be done at all. This would not appear to have been the case with the later Phase II experiments, approved as appropriate at the time, such as those involving children's reaction to radioactive foods or hepatitis. Those studies possibly could have used adults.

So the mere fact that children were involved in the Tudor study is not, alone, basis for adverse ethical or moral judgment.

B. Was There Anything Unethical About the Use of Residents of an Institution?

Participation by institutionalized individuals was approved even after standards were in place during Phase II. For example, the Willowbrook hepatitis study was proposed by a qualified research scientist and approved by the faculty of the NYU School of Medicine, among others. It involved institutionalized children who were mentally retarded. At least the children used in the Tudor study were of normal intelligence. The study involving the injection of cancer cells used institutionalized adults.

Moreover, in 1939, it was totally acceptable to use the very institution used in the Tudor study: the Iowa Soldiers' Orphans' Home. Many other University of Iowa professors and graduate students used the facility in this way. In fact, one of the stuttering study participants is quoted as saying, referring to other studies, "Every week somebody else from the university would come and start testing us for God knows what" (Dyer, 2001).

The Iowa State Board of Control, which oversaw the orphanage, encouraged this research, as did, presumably, the university. So far as is known the Iowa Legislature found nothing in this use of the orphanage to which to object. Permission from the orphanage was required, and was obtained.[15]

All considered, it is hard to fault the study because it involved institutionalized subjects even under today's standards, let alone the standards of its time.

C. Was Informed Consent Not Provided?

After standards were in place, the Atomic Energy Commission did not get informed consent before risking radiation for large populations, nor did the Army or CIA. The 1968 NASA standards *expressly permit* the waiver of informed consent requirements when obtaining consent would interfere with the research.[16] Doctors did not always get the consent of their patients when testing new drugs on them. The Sloan-Kettering doctor did not get the consent of those he injected with cancer.

If "informed consent" had always been required much of the early research in social psychology could not have been done. To measure the impact of group pressure on an unknowing individual necessarily requires *some* deception of the uninformed human subject.[17] Indeed, one can question the extent to which, in 2001, college undergraduates enrolled in psychology classes provided "informed consent" to their participation in graduate students' experiments when their participation was made a condition of undergraduates' credit.

Of course, the 1939 experiment was not a NASA study. But it may very well have met NASA's 1968 standard. That is, like the social psychology studies, Tudor's study would have been very difficult if not impossible if the subjects had been told of its nature.Thus, it is not clear that the Phase I Tudor study, even if judged by the standards of Phase II, would necessarily have been unethical if *no* consent had been obtained.

However, there is reason to believe informed consent *was* provided. It would have been unethical to attempt to obtain the consent of children by negotiating with them directly. An adult needed to be involved. But, by definition, no researcher could obtain the consent of the parents of orphans. The only adult who legally could have given consent on behalf of an institutionalized orphan would have been the administrator of the orphanage. And all indications are that he *did* consent.[18] Thus, for a variety of reasons, it seems inappropriate to criticize the study for a failure to obtain the subjects' consent.

D. Did the Researcher Deliberately Do Permanent Harm?

Ambrose and Yairi, otherwise critical of Tudor's conclusions, assert that Dr. Wendell Johnson and Mary Tudor neither did nor intended any permanent harm.[19] They conclude the procedures used did not, and could not have, caused "stuttering."

Injecting cancer or hepatitis into subjects is deliberately doing known harm. Using LSD on unsuspecting subjects to test its possible utility as a military or intelligence weapon is deliberately doing harm. The Johns Hopkins' human subject's death in 2001 resulted from deliberately doing harm. In 2001, testing the efficacy of new drugs on diseased human subjects by deliberately withholding the remedy from the proportion of them getting placebos risked a measure of harm. In the case of young children in Thailand it was the harm we call AIDS (McNeill, 1998).

If it could be documented that Mary Tudor and Dr. Wendell Johnson knew to a certainty that the study would turn normal speakers into lifelong persons who stutter, an ethical inquiry into their judgment might be warranted. But that is not known. And available evidence compels the opposite conclusion.

The 1939 Tudor study involved speaking to children in a manner and with words still used in 2001 by millions of well-meaning parents who want nothing more than to "improve" their child's disfluency.

The hypothesis being tested was that these well-meaning parents' speech is actually increasing, rather than decreasing, their child's disfluency. But Tudor reasonably could have presumed that whatever conditions might be produced from her four months of intermittent contact would be, if anything, only temporary. At worst, they would be conditions that would promptly respond to therapy.

Dr. Wendell Johnson suffered from his own severe stuttering in 1939, and had a reputation among those who knew him for great kindness and sensitivity, especially with children.[20] He personally experienced every day the emotional pain and frustration of stuttering. He single-mindedly devoted his life to improving his own speech and that of other persons who stutter. It is inconceivable that this man would have permitted any study for which there was even a known *risk* to subjects, let alone a *probability*, of producing lifelong persons who stutter.

Compare this experiment with those Dr. Wendell Johnson, who described himself as "a professional white rat," was subjected to by his professors. As one journalist describes it, he "was hypnotized, psychoanalyzed, prodded with electrodes, and told to sit in cold water to have his tremors recorded. Like Demosthenes, the ancient Greek stutterer, he placed pebbles in his mouth [and] had his dominant arm, the right, placed in a cast to help prove his professor's controversial 'cerebral dominance' theory . . . " (Dyer, 2001).[21]

The passage makes three points. It provides a perspective as to the acceptable range of human subject experimentation in Phase I. It shows Dr. Wendell Johnson's commitment to science and the passion he brought to a lifetime of stuttering research. It also demonstrates the rather dramatic contrast between what he was quite willing to endure himself and what was being tested with Mary Tudor's study.

Finally, note that this 1939 study of the impact of speaking to children involved none of the *approved* physical contact, nuclear radiation, drug-induced behavior modification, exposure to disease, untested pharmaceuticals, or other invasive techniques sometimes used in human subject research *after* ethical standards were in place.

E. How Much Permanent Harm Came from This Brief Experiment?

Were the subjects permanently harmed? All that is available are a journalist's repetition of quotes from the subjects, one of whom was hoping to sue the University of Iowa for a substantial sum of money. And even she acknowledged, at the same time she was working with lawyers to build her case, that she did not stutter during the 45 years of her marriage.

And, of course, "a correlation is not a cause." The subjects undoubtedly had many adverse conditions to deal with before, during, and after their stay in the orphanage. Some had become persons who stutter before the study began. Thus, even if a subject did suffer a speech-related problem as an adult, that alone would not indicate it could be traced in any *causal* way to the study. Moreover, the subject the journalist selected to highlight was one whose fluency actually *improved* during the course of the study.[22]

Accept for the sake of argument two false assumptions (false because the evidence strongly suggests the opposite): (a) there was harm, and (b) a causal relation could be shown between the study's procedures and that harm. Even if both were found to be true, if one is to pass moral judgment on the researcher, one must first confront a considerable additional question, which the passage of time prevents answering: How deliberate or predictable was any of this harm?

This was original research. As discussed above, there was a substantial probability there would be no effect whatsoever on the subjects. The hypothesis, however interesting, might have proven to be totally invalid, as have so many research scientists' hypotheses before and since (and as its critics suggest was the case with the Tudor study).

There is reason to know that the injection of cancer or hepatitis is going to cause temporary or permanent harm. There was no reason to believe that even troublesome temporary, let alone permanent, harm would result from speaking to children in the ways parents do.

It would have been reasonable for the researcher to believe, knowing what was then known, that any disfluencies created in the six subjects' speech during this brief, four-month experiment would quickly disappear.

If in fact disfluencies occurred, and did not disappear in all subjects, it is certainly regrettable. But it does not automatically follow that it represents a reprehensible moral and ethical lapse on the part of the researcher. This is true regardless of whether one evaluates it by the norms of Phase I, when it occurred, or by comparing it with numerous studies done *after* ethical standards were in place during Phase II.

Even had there been known risks, recall today's standard with regard to risks from human subjects research. The standard is not that no risks may be taken. It is, according to the NIH, that risks *not* be taken *unless* "risks to subjects are reasonable relative to . . . the importance of the knowledge that may reasonably be expected to result."

Given the millions of persons who stutter who have benefited from stuttering research, and the millions of children who have *not* become persons who stutter because the findings have been communicated to parents, even if permanent harm could be shown (and apparently it cannot) one could still argue that the NIH standard of permissible risk was met.

As one person who stutters puts the question, and then answers it: "Were the experiments justified? Was their potential benefit to society greater than the potential harm to the subjects? Speaking as a stutterer myself, I think 'yes.' Johnson's results showed that stuttering is learned behavior that can be modified, not a congenital curse that has to be accepted as given. Johnson gave hope and opportunity to the thousands of us who are afflicted with stuttering" (Hedges, 2001, p. 4).

F. Was There a Way of Testing the Tudor Study's Hypothesis Without Involving Children?

Tudor did not have the option of using laboratory or animal studies. Obviously, animal studies are of no use when studying *human* communication. And if the focus of a study is on disfluency in young children, as it was, the participation of young children is required.

The conclusion may be that human subjects research ethics preclude anyone ever finding out what the Tudor study sought to explore. If so, that is a very heavy price to pay. But even that conclusion makes the point. Whatever other ethical criticism is made of the Tudor study, it cannot be faulted for its failure to use an obvious alternative methodology. There simply was none.

G. Were a Large Number of Subjects Affected?

It is regrettable if even one human subject is harmed by a research project. But the fact is that very few subjects were involved in any way in the 1939 Tudor study, especially when compared with the numbers in the Phase II studies. Tens of thousands were potentially involved in the atomic bomb tests. Twelve thousand babies were harmed by thalidomide.

Only two or three of the stuttering research subjects were even *alleged* to have been adversely affected, and that was in support of their quest for legal damages. As discussed above, re-examination of Tudor's data suggests that, not only were no subjects permanently harmed, but given the nature of the experimental design they could not have been.

H. Did the Experiment Continue After the Results Were Known?

The disfluency experiment was a short-lived four-month study. Once the hypothesis was tested and thought to have been strengthened, the study ceased. Compare this ethical response with what was done in the Tuskegee study over the course of not 4 months but 40 years.

Clearly the study cannot be faulted on grounds there was a purposeful, continuing, callous abuse of anyone.

I. Was There Any After-Study Concern for the Subjects?

An effort was made to provide poststudy recuperative therapy for any Tudor subject who might benefit from it. Even Tudor ethics critic Jim Dyer acknowledges that "Johnson asked Tudor to evaluate the children and try to reverse the effects of the experiment using positive therapy" (Dyer, 2001). Judging by the number of subjects who have told the media they suffered no long-term consequences the therapy may well have been helpful.

But this was the dawn of human understanding of speech disfluency and persons who stutter. Therapies that were routine in 2001 were simply unknown at the time. It is not clear that there was anything more that could have been done in 1939. In hindsight, a critic could argue that additional recuperative therapy should have been provided anyway, if for no other reason than to remove any possible question regarding the researcher's desire to be helpful.

The very least that must be credited, however, is that there was far more after-study concern and care of the Tudor subjects than was provided in many human subjects experiments thereafter.

J. Were the Results Not Published and the Data Destroyed?

Some media reported that the results of the Tudor study were never published. Standing alone this is so misleading as to be false.

As with all masters theses at the University of Iowa at the time, the Tudor thesis was bound, given to the University's library, cataloged, and made available to the public. It was often checked out. There was no effort to suppress it.

Few masters theses are commercially published or reprinted in academic journals.[23] They are shelved in academic libraries. That is what was done with this one. It is apparently true that the study was not cited very often in subsequent academic articles.[24] But that is also the fate of much scholarship.

It is not customary to save all the research data associated with a masters thesis. But it is certainly inaccurate to suggest that the data in this study was "destroyed." Not only is it contained within the thesis itself, but some media reports indicate that much if not all of the raw notes were saved, in this instance by the student who did the study.

Making the study available and saving the research data, especially if the researcher and supervisor had any concerns regarding the results, compares very well with, say, the 1973 actions of the CIA director who deliberately destroyed records of the agency's 150 LSD studies.

A responsible, sober analysis of the *elements* of human subjects research ethics, rather than a sensationalist broadside accusation, requires that one ask, "What is it *exactly* about the Tudor study that was unethical?" From that perspective, at a minimum it compares very favorably with an element-by-element analysis of later Phase II studies.

V. Measured by the Standards of Its Time

Given that the Nuremberg Code did not come into existence until 1948, the fact is that there were no international, federal, or state laws, regulations, or other standards applicable to the Tudor study in 1939. As noted earlier, the procedures and ethical standards of the Tudor study researcher were "well within the norms of the time."

The most rational and fair approach is to judge the ethics of the study by the research standards of the time, nationally, in Iowa, at the University of Iowa, and at the institution where the subjects lived. By those standards it seems somewhere between very difficult and impossible to come to any critical ethical judgment.

Indeed, what is particularly striking, given the absence of standards, is the sensitivity both the researcher and supervisor brought to the subjects of the study, self-imposed standards that compare very favorably with those of 2001.

VI. Measured by the Standards of 2001

As mentioned above, it seems no more appropriate to judge the ethics of actions in 1939 by the standards of 2001 than to later pass ethical judgment on our 2001 behavior from the vantage point of the ethical standards of 2063.[25]

Many of the Tudor study's critics have fallen into a trap well known to general semanticists.[26] These critics think and speak as if "ethics is ethics." General semanticists use what they call "dates and indexes." They are never surprised to find, indeed they rather expect, that "ethics1939" is not at all like "ethics2001."

As the previous section has demonstrated, however, even if one uses the totally inappropriate standards of 2001, the Phase I Tudor study still appears more ethical than many of the studies going on in Phase IV, not to mention Phases II and III.

It may turn out that no one has yet earned the right to cast moral aspersions on those whose pioneering work was done 62 years earlier. After all the pious proclamations from the Tudor study's self-righteous critics, and their insistence the human species has evolved into creatures with a much heightened ethical and moral sense, things still are far from perfect in research land.

The evolution of human morality and ethics with regard to any aspect of human behavior is usually a very slow process.[27] Moreover, even with standards in place the mere existence of institutions, regulations, and ethical standards seldom proves to be enough to protect the rights of human subjects, as the following examples demonstrate.

A 1994 Department of Energy advisory committee report contains an historical account of Public Health Service employees' site visits to research institutions. Those visits "revealed a wide range of compliance . . . confusion about how to assess risks and benefits, refusal by some researchers to cooperate with the [PHS] policy, and in many cases, indifference by those charged with administering research and its rules at local institutions."

As late as the post-1998 period the NIH shut down research programs at eight prestigious institutions for a variety of ethical violations. They included the September 1999 death of a human subject in a gene therapy study who, it is alleged, was not adequately informed of the risks.

Consider the April 2000 report of the DHHS Office of Inspector General, "Protecting Human Research Subjects." The report notes the office's concerns two years earlier: a "call for widespread reform," "a sense of urgency," "disturbing inadequacies in IRB oversight of clinical trials," up to and including "the death of a teenager participating in a gene transfer clinical trial funded by NIH."

Presumably death could be considered a kind of "permanent harm" at least the equivalent of children's speech disfluency.

Notwithstanding these concerns, the report noted, "few of [the office's] recommended reforms have been enacted." IRBs are focusing "on review responsibilities of questionable protective value" while giving low priority to protecting human subjects. Many IRBs give reviews insufficient attention, and subsequently "know little of what actually occurs." Many researchers are untrained in human subjects research standards because "No educational requirements have been enacted." Increased commercialization in studies was a concern because it "heightens the potential for conflicts of interest in clinical research."

As late as October 2000 the NIH was still sufficiently concerned about researchers' lack of knowledge, understanding, and compliance with human research standards that it began to require proof of the education of researchers regarding those standards before studies are funded and undertaken.

Some of the ethical practices used by U.S. institutions with their research in developing countries could well be subject to serious criticism. One example may be enough to make the point.

A major academic journal reported in March 2000 a study reminiscent of the Tuskegee syphilis study (Quinn, 2000). It was done by researchers from no less prestigious a research institution than Johns Hopkins. In the Rakai region of Uganda they monitored 415 couples, of which only one partner was infected with HIV. The researchers did not inform the AIDS-free partners. Thirty months later 90 of the formerly healthy spouses had become infected. The journal's editor noted that the study was unethical by U.S. standards.

In July 2001 there were news reports that the federal Office for Human Research Protections had shut down human subjects research at Johns Hopkins. This was huge; all Hopkins medical institutions combined received $419 million in research funds from the NIH alone in 2000, the most of any such institution. The cited reason? "This is about protecting people's lives." The precipitating cause? The death of yet another human subject.[28]

The contrast between the media's coverage of this 2001 death at one of the nation's largest research institutions and the coverage of the little 1939 Tudor study is striking. The word "hypocrisy" may or may not be misplaced, but "disparity" certainly is not.

There were no editorials passing moral judgment on the Hopkins researchers and their institution. No characterization of their work as a "monster study." No calls for punishment, or for removing names from buildings. Indeed, there was not even an editorial demand for apologies to the family members of the dead subject, let alone proposals that they be paid damages, all of which at least some editors thought appropriate for the 1939 study. There were no known media mentions of expressions of sympathy or sorrow for the deceased's survivors, though surely there must have been some. Table 9-1 compares the two studies.

Table 9–1. The 1939 Tudor Masters Thesis Versus The 2001 Hopkins Study

The 1939 Tudor Masters Thesis	The 2001 Johns Hopkins Study
The 1939 study was conducted before any ethical standards were in place; before even the Nuremberg and Helsinki statements. All possible standards were violated. No approvals were obtained.	The 2001 study was conducted after decades of evolution of detailed, written ethical standards. Those standards were violated. Yet the relevant IRB approved the study.
The 1939 study involved a young masters degree student with little or no funding, staff, or research experience.	The Johns Hopkins study involved respected professionals in the largest medical research institution in the country (the recipient of $419 million for taxpayer-supported research).
The 1939 study was conducted before there was any way of knowing what impact it would have upon the subjects, and every reason to believe any adverse effects easily could be reversed. It was original research; by definition there was no prior literature.	The Hopkins study involved the use of hexamethonium, a chemical about which much was known and published. It was known to cause lung damage, which was why it was used. It was given in amounts characterized as "extraordinarily large"; amounts the FDA would not have approved had it been asked.

Continued

Table 9–1. *Continued*

The 1939 Tudor Masters Thesis	The 2001 Johns Hopkins Study
The 1939 study involved the maximum informed consent possible (that of the adult administrator of the children's institution). No objections were raised to the study from the university, the institution, or the state agency with oversight responsibility. The researcher complied fully with the informed consent required by the ethical standards of the time.	The 2001 study's subjects provided a measure of consent, but it was not fully informed, as required. They were unaware of the full extent of the risks to which they were being subjected—such as death from the total destruction of their lungs. What they were told was a "medication"—was in fact a lung irritant, not an asthma remedy. The chemical had lost FDA approval for its original purpose in 1972, was not FDA-approved for this study, was used experimentally, in excessive amounts, and had never been approved in an inhaled form.
The 1939 study is criticized because the researcher's speaking to the subjects in ways millions of parents did in 2001 did not involve the evaluation of a *cure* for stuttering. There were no "cures" for stuttering to be tested in 1939.	There *were* possible cures for asthma in 2001. Yet in researching asthma the Hopkins researcher deliberately used a chemical he knew would *worsen* the subjects' lung condition. The study was in no sense a search for a "cure."
The 1939 study is criticized (falsely according to the best data) for causing permanent disfluency in the subjects.	The 2001 study caused a death, surely a kind of permanent harm the full equivalent of disfluency, even if not in the minds of many journalists and editorial writers.
The very least that can be said is that the 1939 researcher did not knowingly and deliberately do permanent harm to the subjects.	The 2001 researcher either knew, or ought to have known (based on the required literature search), that his deliberate actions risked permanent harm, including death, to his subjects. Indeed, his description of the study said its purpose was "to find out how the tubes that carry air into the lungs can stay open even when we breathe all types of irritating chemicals." This was, by any definition, knowingly and deliberately doing harm.

Whatever may be said by way of criticism of the ethics of the Tudor study, any fair critic would have to concede that, even applying the ethical standards of 2001, it compares very favorably to the studies to which those ethical standards clearly *do* apply.

VII. Scholarship and Scandals

A. Why Select the Tudor Study for Ethical Analysis?

There is a legitimate academic interest in the theories being tested by the Tudor study and the impact of those theories, and Tudor's evidence, on the history of stuttering research and therapy which followed. That is the focus of much of this book.

Moreover, human subjects research ethics, and the evolution of the standards reflecting those moral principles and ethical practices, are also clearly important subjects worthy of academic, and even journalistic, attention.

But *if* one is going to pursue an inquiry into human subjects research generally, there is a very large, and as yet unanswered, question as to why the Tudor study would play *any* role. Singling out Tudor as *the* case study in such an inquiry is, at best, a little bizarre.

Reflect on the thousands of studies that have been conceived, reviewed, approved, funded, and carried out by academic research institutions during the last half of the twentieth century, some of which are detailed in section II. D., above. Obviously, many prominent and reputable academic researchers, institutions, and granting agencies believed that those studies were defensible *after* ethical standards were in place.

By what logic would one ignore *those* studies? Why would one stretch to single out for moral judgment a little 1939 masters thesis, conceived and carried out long before any such standards existed?

B. Why Would University and Association Officers Join in the Critical Chorus?

Why would an officer of a professional association that includes speech-language pathologists want to say, not incidentally of a person involved in the early years of that association, that the Tudor research "cannot be justified on theoretical, moral or ethical grounds and represented a serious error of judgment" (Bernthal, 2001)?

Why would a current university administrator at Dr. Wendell Johnson's institution want to be quoted as saying, "This is not a study that should ever be considered defensible in any era. In no way would I ever think of defending this study. In no way. It's more than unfortunate" (Ratliff, 2001)?[29]

It may be "more than unfortunate" that the mass media brought the Tudor study to national attention. But if it was so indefensible, if castigation and apologies are so necessary, why was none of this said and done when the study was spread across a local newspaper in that university's town years ago, described in an academic journal years before that, and subsequently found its way into a novel?[30]

The university administrator and association officer quoted above were unwavering in their rectitude. "The University of Iowa today has in place a strict policy and procedures [so that] experiments of this nature [the Tudor study] cannot happen again," says one (Jacobson, 2001, p. 1A).[31] "Such research is strictly prohibited under [the association's] Code of Ethics," says the other (Bernthal, 2001).

They thereby built themselves a very high pulpit from which to cast moral judgments on their predecessors below. Unfortunately, it sat atop a shaky scaffolding from which their fall from grace proved to be as prompt as it was painful. Not only were there the numerous examples of unethical practices throughout the research community in 2001, detailed in section V., above, but the University of Iowa in particular found itself criticized for its own violations less than a week after the Hopkins death was reported.[32]

Is this but one more example of a professional association and research institution primarily responding to the public relations demands[33] of a negative national media blitz? Or is there evidence of genuine concern for the subjects and the ethical issues involved?

C. The Ethical Failures of the Ethical Criticism

Such moral castigation, and the tabloid-style journalism that preceded and provoked it, have the effect of removing the Tudor study from meaningful perspective.

They fail to place the Tudor study within a context of the decades-long body of speech pathology research; to describe for persons who stutter, and the parents of those to come, the array of available assistance[34]; or the historical evolution of human subjects research ethics, which cannot be explained with sound bites and knee-jerk moral judgments. And they fail to recognize the place of the Tudor study in the lifetime body of stuttering research at the University of Iowa in general and of Dr. Wendell Johnson in particular (Johnson, 1930; Johnson, 1946; Johnson, 1955; Johnson, 1959; Moeller, 1975).[35]

It might be worth the price of tarnishing the reputation of a highly respected scientist, even a deceased giant from one's own institution, if it could contribute to a substantial improvement in public policy.

But comments and articles about the Tudor study are unlikely to have much, if any, impact on evolving human subjects research ethical standards and their administration.[36] Indeed, it truly would be shocking if a 62-year-old, Phase I masters thesis could raise ethical issues that had been neither recognized nor addressed in the detailed Phase IV regulations in place by 2001.

It also might be worth harming a reputation if the revelations would help millions, thousands, hundreds, or even dozens of people. There are numerous examples in which that is the case, involving everything from information about tobacco, asbestos, and pharmaceuticals' side effects to silicone breast implants and environmental lead and mercury.

It is not clear whether *any* of the Tudor subjects were harmed by the study in any way. Worst case, which requires that the assertions of litigants and their lawyers be treated as fact rather than negotiating gambits, there were one or two individuals whose disfluency increased.

The question is not whether a mere two people matter. Of course they do. The question is whether the publication of these articles and administrators' comments in 2001 did not do even *them* more harm than good.

D. Journalist Heal Thyself

It is pointless to speculate as to a journalist's motives. It does appear that there was a deliberate dramatization of a 62-year-old masters thesis into a national story discrediting the reputations of the researcher and a supervisor 36-years dead.

This is the stuff for which the law provides remedies, such as defamation or false light. They involve a defendant's use of a fact here and there to present a false and damaging impression of someone.

The author of the newspaper stories in question was quick to cast moral opprobrium on the researcher and supervisor of the Tudor study. He was considerably slower in coming to an examination of his own ethical lapses. In fact, it appears he never bothered to consider them at all.

Journalistic ethics is not the oxymoron some may believe it to be.[37] There is a Society of Professional Journalists, which has created a "Code of Ethics." By 2001 the most recent version of the Code was the one adopted in September 1996 (Society of Professional Journalists, 1996). There are a number of provisions in this Code that raise issues with regard to the ethics of the reporter's and newspaper's handling and promotion of their stories about the Tudor study.

The Code speaks of goals such as "public enlightenment" from journalism. It says that journalists have a "duty" to "further those ends by . . . providing a fair and comprehensive account of . . . issues . . . [and] to serve the public with thoroughness and honesty." They "should . . . examine their own cultural values and avoid imposing those values on others."

Journalists should "show compassion to those who may be affected adversely by news coverage . . . recognize that gathering and reporting information may cause harm or discomfort . . . [and] that private people have a greater right to control information about themselves than do public officials. . . . Only an overriding public need can justify intrusion into anyone's privacy."

Finally, in a Code provision perhaps more applicable to editors than reporters, "Journalists should . . . make certain that headlines, news teases and promotional material, photos, video, audio, graphics, sound bites and quotations do not misrepresent. They should not oversimplify or highlight incidents out of context."

Consider the actions of Dyer and the *Mercury News* when measured by the standards of these admonitions.

The *Mercury News'* stories detracted from, rather than added to, "public enlightenment" about ethics in human subjects research in general and the ethics of the Tudor study in particular. Their account of the issues was neither "fair and comprehensive" nor presented with "thoroughness and honesty."

One of the more serious indictments of the journalist's professional ethics and abilities is that the very human subject he selected to highlight was one whose fluency actually *improved* during the course of the study.[38] Whatever this may indicate regarding the validity of the theory drawn from the data by the researcher, it certainly seriously undercuts the journalist's efforts to trash the reputations of Dr. Wendell Johnson and Mary Tudor because of the harm he alleges they did to the subjects. One would think that a "fair" account, presented with "honesty" would require, at a minimum, a measure of factual accuracy. The journalist may have been unaware of his ethical transgression. Perhaps he did it deliberately. Or maybe it was simply a sloppy job of research and writing. And which would be worse?

The journalist failed to heed the ethical requirement that he "avoid imposing [his cultural] values on others;" moreover, in this case others who lived and acted in a different time and place, 62 years before the story was written. He failed to "show compassion to those who may be affected adversely by news coverage." There was no demonstration of compassion, and total indifference to "information [that] may cause harm or discomfort" to the named subjects, the researcher, and the family survivors of the supervisor of the study.

There was no apparent "overriding public need [to] justify intrusion into anyone's privacy." In order to avoid invasions of privacy at least the researcher had exercised enough sensitivity to refer to the subjects only by number rather than by name. Unfortunately, the journalist chose to ignore both the *researcher's* sense of decency and *his* ethical responsibilities.

The journalists' Code of Ethics also provides that, "Journalists should . . . avoid undercover or other surreptitious methods of gathering information except when traditional open methods will not yield information vital to the public. Use of such methods should be explained as part of the story."

On July 25, 2001, the journalist's executive editor felt obliged to run an editorial revealing that the journalist had violated the paper's own ethical standards regarding "surreptitious methods" (a provision equivalent to that quoted above).[39] The journalist had gained entry to a State of Iowa archive that is closed to journalists. He had misrepresented that his role was that of an academic researcher. The editor failed to mention any of the reporter's other ethical violations, including the violation of the privacy rights of the subjects, which was one of the reasons for excluding journalists from the archives.

As for the ethics of the promotional material, consider this promo in the journalist's paper a couple days before the series was scheduled to run. The headline blared:

"San Jose Mercury News Uncovers Secret Experiment to Make Orphans Stutter; Traces Living Legacy of Tormented Children and Haunted Researcher"

The promo began, "In a chilling investigative series beginning Sunday, the Mercury News reveals for the first time the complete story of a secret experiment conducted 60 years ago to induce a group of orphans to stutter. The study [was] designed and concealed by Wendell Johnson . . . "[40]

Consider the inaccuracies and exaggerations. The researcher did not "torment" the subjects. A "haunted" researcher? A "chilling" series? There was nothing to "uncover." The study was not "revealed for the first time." It had been written about by others, including Dyer himself nine years earlier.[41] It was not "a secret experiment." It was not "conducted . . . to induce a group of orphans to stutter." It was not "concealed."

Compare this promotion with the ethical standard. Are these "headlines, news teases and promotional material [that] do not misrepresent; [that do] not oversimplify or highlight incidents out of context"? Or do they (and the series itself) have more in common with sensationalist, tabloid, supermarket scandal sheets?

The journalist's ethical violations ultimately led to his "resignation" (Associated Press, 2001).

It is beyond the scope of this chapter to explore whether he also may have been guilty of defamation or false light. It is enough to note that he is in a very weak position when questioning the ethics of others, especially when he is doing so in the emotionally laden vocabulary of the tabloids. After all, those he criticized acted *before* the existence of relevant ethical standards for human subjects research. He was writing *after* the journalistic ethical standards he violated were in place and applicable to his journalism.

One need not look back on his actions with the benefit of hindsight and judge him by the standards of journalistic ethics 62 years later, in 2063. It is enough to judge him by the standards in place at the time he wrote, standards that presumably were, or ought to have been, well known to him.

VIII. Conclusion

Whatever the Tudor study's *substantive* faults may be, its ethics compare very favorably not only to the standards of its own time, in 1939, but to those of 2001 as well.

If its substantive critics are right, no harm was done or intended, either by Dr. Wendell Johnson or by Mary Tudor. The study could not, and did not, "cause stuttering."

Even if those critics are wrong, and contrary to the best evidence the subjects *did* experience increased disfluency in later life, there is no indication it was *caused* by anything done by Mary Tudor, as distinguished from the subjects' experiences before, during, or after their stay in the institution.

Make three *false* assumptions. Critics of the Tudor study's substance are wrong. The subjects have suffered permanent harm. There is proof beyond a shadow of a doubt that the sole cause of that harm was the Tudor study. Even if each of those false assumptions were true, there still would have been no violations of international or other ethical standards for human subjects research applicable to the Tudor study in 1939. There simply were none in existence at the time.

Even if *all* the above were true, *and* it were to be irrationally and unfairly decided that the study's ethics should be judged by the standards of 2001, it would still be difficult to find serious ethical violations.

One cannot judge the ethics of "the study," only the *specific* ethical standards that are alleged to have been violated. Few, if any, can be found.

Finally, insofar as there might be found to be any specific violations, there are many more, of much greater seriousness, going on today that have *not* brought forth anything like the moral castigation hurled at Dr. Wendell Johnson and Mary Tudor.

So why were the ethics of the Tudor study attacked? This review of the ethics of administration, journalism, and human subjects research provides no answer. And speculation regarding the motives of others is a task even less rewarding than looking for ethical needles in a 62-year-old haystack.

References

Advisory Committee on Human Radiation Experiments Report. Part I, Chapter 3, NASA Policy. Available from: http://www.eh.doe.gov/ohre/roadmap/achre/chap3_3.html

AllAfrica Global Media, "Ethics of Medical Research in the Third World," February 2, 2001. Available from: http://allafrica.com/stories/200102020128.html (requires subscription).

Ambrose, N. G., & Yairi, E. (2002). The Tudor study: Data and ethics. *American Journal of Speech-Language Pathology, 11*, 190–203.

An unnecessary death; Hopkins study: Tighter controls on human research projects needed; institution's inquiry finds faults. (2001, July 18). *The Baltimore Sun.*

Associated Press. (2001, July 31). Stutter story reporter quits. *Iowa City Press-Citizen.*

Associated Press. (2002, December 2). Ore. gov. apologizes for sterilization.

Associated Press. (2005a, May 5). Feds tested AIDS drugs on foster kids.

Associated Press. (2005b, May 18). Deaths prompt end to breast cancer study.

Associated Press. (2005c, May 19). Use of foster kids in experiments varies.

Author of stuttering series quits paper; reporter criticized for research method. (2001, August 1). *Iowa City Gazette*, p. 8A.

Bernthal, J. (2001, June 19). U of I speech study was unethical. *Des Moines Register*, p. 8.

Birch, D. M., & Cohn, G. (2001, June 25). The changing creed of Hopkins science; what once was heresy is now the mission: A partnership with business to advance research. *The Baltimore Sun.*

Bor, J. (2001, June 23). Hopkins panel to study death of volunteer. *The Baltimore Sun.*

Bor, J., & Pelton, T. (2001, June 22). Hopkins study was exempt from FDA; asthma project tested function of lungs, wasn't a drug trial. *The Baltimore Sun.*

Bor, J., & Pelton, T. (2001, July 20). U.S. halts Hopkins research; most experiments on human subjects ordered suspended; federal funding withheld; oversight agency decries safety lapses in volunteer's death. *The Baltimore Sun.*

Carlson, J. (2001, July 17) . U of I, state owe yesteryear's orphans the whole truth. *Des Moines Register*, p. 1B.

The Centers for Disease Control and Prevention. Human subjects research. Available from: http://www.cdc.gov/od/ads/hsr2.htm

Council for International Organizations of Medical Sciences (CIOMS). (1991). International guidelines for ethical review of epidemiological studies (Geneva). Available from: http://www.cdc.gov/od/ads/intlgui3.htm

Death at research center; Hopkins study: Volunteer's death raises questions about protection, role of human research aubjects. (2002, July 1). *The Baltimore Sun.*

Defense department. offers details of toxic tests done in secret. (2001, October 10). *New York Times.*

Department of Energy's Advisory Committee on Human Radiation Experiments Report. DOE openness: Human radiation experiments. Available from: http://tis.eh.doe.gov/ohre/roadmap/achre/

Department of Health and Human Services' Office for Human Research Protections. Available from: http://www.hhs.gov/ohrp/

Department of Health and Human Services' Office for Human Research Protections. Educational material for researchers. Available from: http://www.hhs.gov/ohrp/education/index.html#materials

Department of Health and Human Services, Office of Inspector General. (2000, April). Protecting human research subjects. Available from: http://www.oig.hhs.gov/oei/reports/oei-01-97-00197.pdf

Drew, G. (n.d.). Side-by-side comparison of 1996 and 2000 declaration of Helsinki. Available from: http://www.hhs.gov/ohrp/nhrpac/mtg12-00/h1996-2000.pdf

Dyer, J. (1992, April). The twisted experiment of Dr. Wendell Johnson. *The Iowa City Mercury*, p. 1.

Dyer, J. (2001, June 10). Ethics and orphans: The monster study. Part one of a Mercury News Special Report. *San Jose [CA] Mercury News*, p. 1A.

Dyer, J. (2001, June 11). Ethics and orphans: The Monster Study. Part two of a Mercury News Special Report. *San Jose [CA] Mercury News*, p. 1A.

Eberlein, T. J. (2000, February 17). Medical insurers should pay for clinical trials of experimental cancer treatments. Washington University St. Louis *Record*. Available from: http://wupa.wustl.edu/record/archive/2000/02-17-00/articles/eberlein.html

178   ETHICS: A CASE STUDY

Egan, G., Jones, R., & Ranvaud, D. (Producers), & Meirelles, F. (Director). (2005). *The constant gardener* [Movie]. United States: Paramount.

FDA Backgrounder. (n.d.) Milestones in U.S. food and drug law history; Kefauver-Harris drug amendments of 1962. Available from: http://www.cfsan.fda.gov/mileston.html

Flaum, M. (2002, September 4). Research did not cause stuttering. Guest opinion. *The Daily Iowan*, p. 8A.

Foley, R. (2001, July 26). "Monster study" reporter under fire. *The Daily Iowan*, p. 1.

Fraser, J. (2001, July 10). *The Fresno Bee*, p. B6.

Halvorson, J. (1999). *Abandoned: Now stutter my orphan.* Hagar City, IA: Halvorson Farms of Wisconsin.

Hedges, J. (2001, June 25). A new perspective on stuttering research. *The Daily Iowan*, p. 4.

Hilts, P. J. (2001, August 21). Drug's problems raise questions on warnings. *New York Times*.

Hinman, L. M. (n.d.) University of San Diego, Ethics updates. Available from: http://ethics.acusd.edu/

Hopkins calls federal agency's action "precipitous." (2001, July 20). *The Baltimore Sun*.

Jacobson, J. (2001, June 13). UI denounces experiment. *Iowa City Gazette*, p. 1A.

Jacobson, J. (2001, July 21). UI funding unaffected by halt in Johns Hopkins cancer study. *Iowa City Gazette*, p. 1.

Johnson, N. Psychology's special problems. In: Cites, sites, sources and notes. Available as a link from: www.nicholasjohnson.org

Johnson, N. Wendell A. L. Johnson memorial home page. Available as a link from: http://www.nicholasjohnson.org

Johnson, W. (1930). *Because I stutter.* New York: Appleton.

Johnson, W. (1946). *People in quandaries.* New York: Harper & Brothers.

Johnson, W. (Ed.). (1955). *Stuttering in children and adults.* Minneapolis: University of Minnesota Press.

Johnson, W. (Ed.). (1959). *The onset of stuttering: Research findings and implications.* Minneapolis: University of Minnesota Press.

Journals adopt new policy: Editors aim to clip drug companies' influence. (2001, August 5). *Iowa City Press-Citizen*, p. 1A.

Knabe, J., Gingerich, P., Fesenmeyer, N., Lorack J., & Hubbard, B. (2001, July 5). Wendell Johnson was a fine man: Judge him in light of the times. *Iowa City Gazette*, p. 7A.

Kolata, G. (2001, July 20). U.S. suspends human research at Johns Hopkins after a death. *New York Times*.

Krantz, C. (2001, June 14). U of I rues experiment on stutterers. *Des Moines Register*, p. 1.

Krantz, C. (2001, July 9). "Orphans Targeted for Tests." *Des Moines Register*, p. 1.

Krantz, C. (2001, July 22). U of I faces probe over research. *Des Moines Sunday Register*, p. 1.

LeCarré, John. (2001). *The constant gardener.* New York: Scribner.

McBride, K. (2004). Journalists: More ethical than people realize?, *Poynteronline*. Available from http://www.poynter.org/content/content_print.asp?id=75962&custom=

McNeill, P. M. (1998). Should research ethics change at the border? *The Medical Journal of Australia, 169,* 509–510. Available from: http://www.mja.com.au/public/issues/nov16/mcneill/mcneill.html

Medical journals battle drug firms' grip on research. (2001, August 5). *Iowa City Gazette*, p. 3A.

Mercury News. (2004, September 24). Ethics policy. Available from: http://www.grandforks.com/mld/mercurynews/contact_us/about/9723906.htm

Milisen, R. L. (2001, July 27). Johnson was a great man. *Iowa City Press-Citizen*, p. 11A.

Mitchell, G. (2004, December 7). Reporters trail badly (again) in annual poll on honesty and ethics. Available from: http://www.editorandpublisher.com/eandp/news/article_display.jsp?vnu_content_id=1000732750

Moeller, D. (1975). *Speech pathology and audiology: Iowa origins of a discipline* (pp. 61–62). Iowa City: University of Iowa.

The National Commission for the Protection of Human Subjects of Biomedical and Behavioral Research. (1979, April 18). Ethical principles and guidelines for the protection of human subjects of research (The Belmont report). Available from: http://www.hhs.gov/ohrp/humansubjects/guidance/belmont.htm

National Institute of Health, Office of Human Subjects Research. (n.d.). Criteria for institutional review board (IRB) approval of research involving human subjects. Available from: http://www.nihtraining.com/ohsrsite/info/sheet3.html

The National Library of Medicine. (n.d.). Current bibliographies in medicine: Ethical issues in research involving human participants. *Current Bibliographies in Medicine*, 99-3. Available from: http://www.nlm.nih.gov/pubs/cbm/hum_exp.html

National Public Radio. (2001, June 23). Weekly edition.

Of profits and patients; medical research: Academic institutions face huge conflicts of interest as they pursue business ties. (2001, July 2). *The Baltimore Sun.*

Okie, S. (2001, August 5). A stand for scientific independence: Medical journals aim to curtail drug companies' influence. *Washington Post*, p. A1.

Pappas, G. (2001, July 23). Gov't probe of UI research "minor." *The Daily Iowan*, p. 1.

Pappas, G. (2001, July 24). UI fires back at register's headline. *The Daily Iowan*, p. 1.

Pelton, T. (2001, July 3). Asthma study violated safety rules, FDA says; Hopkins experiment ended with death of volunteer, 24. *The Baltimore Sun*.

Pelton, T. (2001, July 8). Respected doctors confront a tragedy; experiment: With a research subject's death, two distinguished scientists confront what colleagues say is the worst imaginable outcome. *The Baltimore Sun*.

Pelton, T., & Bor, J. (2001, July 21). Hopkins vows to improve research safety; changes outlined in letter school sent to federal agency; "It's Been Utter Confusion;" lifting of suspension sought by next week. *The Baltimore Sun*.

PETA (People for the Ethical Treatment of Animals). (n.d.). Available from: http://www.peta.org

PETA, (n.d.). Cruel science. Available from: http://www.peta.org/cmp/sci.html

Protecting humans in research; Hopkins shutdown: Government is right to be concerned, but wrong to punish researchers so harshly. (2001, July 21). *The Baltimore Sun*.

Quinn, T. C. (2000). Viral load and heterosexual transmission of human immunodeficiency virus Type 1. *New England Journal of Medicine*, 342, 921–929.

Quesal, R.W. (2001). Personal communication.

Ratliff, K. (2001, June 12). UI stuttering study doubted. *Iowa City Press-Citizen*, pp. 1, 7.

Ratliff, K. (2001, June 14). UI apologizes for research on stuttering. *Iowa City Press-Citizen*, p. 1A.

Shea, C. (2000). Don't talk to the humans. *Linguafranca*, 10.

Siegel E., & Sugg, D. K. (2001, June 24). Management of crisis key to public trust. *The Baltimore Sun*.

Silverman, E-M. (2001, June 18). Paper missed chance to better inform readers. *Milwaukee Journal Sentinel*, p. 10A.

Silverman, F. (1988). The monster study. *Journal of Fluency Disorders*, 13, 225–231.

Skorton, D. (2001, August 5). No action pending regarding U of I research. [Opinion.] *Des Moines Register*, p. 9A.

Society of Professional Journalists. (1996). Code of ethics. Available from: http://www.spj.org/ethics_code.asp

Spielman, M. Z. (2005, February 25). U.S. journalists get high marks on ethics, study finds; LSU and University of Missouri professors analyze the "moral minds" of journalists and advertisers. *LSU's Biweekly*

Newsletter for Faculty & Staff, 21. Available from: http://www.lsu. edu/lsutoday/050225/pageone.html

Stanford University. (n.d.). Use of human subjects in research: History. Avalable from: http://www.stanford.edu/department/DoR/hs/ History/his01.html

John, R., & Stanley, J. R. (2000). Ethical accusations: The loss of common sense. *Archives of Dermatology, 136,* 268–269. Available from: http://archderm.ama-assn.org/cgi/content/extract/136/2/268-a

Stewart, J. L. (1992–93). Wendell Johnson: A memoir. *Et cetera,* p. 424.

Stop Animal Tests. Available from: http://www.stopanimaltests.com

Stroh, M. (2001, July 20). Shutdowns have wide effect on programs; cutting-edge treatments become unavailable; funding, name damaged. *The Baltimore Sun.*

Sugg, D. K. (2001, July 21). Despite suspension, Hopkins researchers continue vital tests; doctors, nurses rush to reassure patients, appeal research bans. *The Baltimore Sun.*

Trials of war criminals before the Nuremberg military tribunals under control council law, 1949. *Nuremberg code: Directives for human experimentation,* 2(10), 181–182. Washington, DC: U.S. Government Printing Office. Available from: http://ohsr.od.nih.gov/guidelines/ nuremberg.html.

Tudor, M. (1939). *An experimental study of the effect of evaluative labeling on speech fluency.* Unpublished master's thesis, University of Iowa, Iowa City.

UI apologizes for stuttering study. (2001, June 14). *San Jose Mercury News.*

United Nations. (1948). Declaration of human rights. Available from http://un.org/Overview/rights.htm

University apologizes for '39 experiment. (2001, June 14). *Chicago Tribune,* p. 19.

University of Michigan. (n.d.). Protection of human research subjects computer-based training for researchers. See The National Cancer Institute, Human participant protections education for research teams. Available from: http://cme.cancer.gov/clinicaltrials/learning/ humanparticipant-protections.asp

The Virginia Commonwealth University. (n.d.). Ethics of research involving human participation. Available from: http://www.vcu. edu/hasweb/psy/faculty/fors/ethics.htm

Williams, D. (1992–93, Winter). Remembering Wendell Johnson. *Et cetera,* p. 433. [Reprinted from the May 4, 1992 issue of the *Daily Iowan*].

Wise, P. (2001, June 8). Press release, *Mercury News.*

World Health Organization. (n.d.). Ethics and health. Available from: http://www.who.int [click on Research Ethics].

World Health Organization. (2002). International ethical guidelines for biomedical research involving human subjects. Available from:

http://www.who.int/bookorders/anglais/detart1.jsp?sesslan=1&c
odlan=1&codcol=84&codcch=2016

World Medical Association. (1964–2000). World Medical Association
(WMA) declaration of Helsinki ethical principles for medical
research involving human subjects (Declaration of Helsinki).
Adopted by the 18th WMA, Helsinki, Finland, June 1964, and
amended by the 29th WMA, Tokyo, Japan, October, 1975, 35th
WMA, Venice, Italy, October 1983, 41st WMA, Hong Kong, Septem-
ber 1989, 48th WMA General Assembly, Somerset west, Republic of
South Africa, October 1996, and the 52nd WMA General Assembly,
Edinburgh, Scotland, October 2000. Available from: http://www.
nihtraining.com/ohsrsite/guidelines/helsinki.html

Yarnold, D. (2001, July 25). Setting the record straight. *The San Jose
Mercury News*.

Endnotes

1. This chapter is supported by a Web site at http://www. nicholasjohnson.org. Many of the chapter's citations are to on-line material. Although the URL links were working when the book went to press, in the future some may no longer function. Thus, the Web site provides updated URLs. It also contains links to the original version of this chapter presented as a paper, additional references beyond those listed here, the Wendell A.L. Johnson Memorial Home Page, and additional information about the author.

This chapter only addresses the ethical issues surrounding the Tudor study. It leaves to research scientists' other chapters the analysis of the Tudor study data and conclusions. It presumes the reader has at least some awareness of stuttering research in general, the research of Dr. Wendell Johnson in particular, and most especially a 1939 masters thesis by one of his graduate students, Mary Tudor.

2. The emotionally-loaded quality of the reporting is illustrated by the language used in the accompanying promotion:

> [In the] 'Monster Study' in 1939, an ambitious professor conducted a secret experiment on a group of orphans to test a new theory on stuttering. The results helped gain renown for the professor, but many of the children were psychologically harmed for life. The study was covered up, even from the orphans—until now.

Aside from the obvious difficulties one would confront in an effort to "gain renown" from a "secret experiment" that was "covered up . . . until now"—even one known to be a "monster study"—the numerous violations of journalistic ethics represented by the newspaper's stories and promotional announcements are detailed in section VII. D., in the text.

There is no evidence for the assertions that the study, often examined by researchers and referenced in print (including an earlier story by this very reporter), was "covered up . . . until now," that it involved "stuttering" rather than "disfluency," or that "many of the children were psychologically harmed for life."

Part Two was published by the same newspaper June 11, 2001, also on page 1A. Its promotional material included this quote: "An experiment leaves a lifetime of anguish [as] the study's young victims were left in ignorance, to cope alone. Experts debate whether the benefits justified the harm."

3. "For [former University of Iowa Vice President for Research] Duane Spriestersbach . . . [the] experiment was both justified and ethical. 'It was a different time and the values were different. . . . Today we might disagree with what he did, but in those days it was fully within the norms of the time.'" Jim Dyer, "Ethics and Orphans: The Monster Study," Part Two of a Mercury News Special Report, *San Jose* [CA] *Mercury News*, June 11, 2001, p. 1A. Others agree. "The University of Iowa's stuttering experiment six decades ago . . . wouldn't have been considered so unusual at the time, according to experts." Colleen Krantz, "Orphans Targteted for Tests," *Des Moines Register*, July 9, 2001, p. 1. As then-University of Iowa President Mary Sue Coleman put it, "It was a different time and place." Jim Jacobson, "UI Denounces Experiment," *Iowa City Gazette*, June 13, 2001, p. 1A. The University's Human Subjects Office director, Trish Wasek, said, "It was a different time and a different set of mores in existence at the time." Colleen Krantz, "U of I Rues Experiment on Stutterers," *Des Moines Register*, June 14, 2001, p. 1.

4. That this is not always the case, that there are mature adult responses occasionally, is illustrated by the *Baltimore Sun*'s noting the contrast between the responses of Johns Hopkins and Rochester researchers after the death of a human subject. "In Rochester in 1996 [following the death of a human subject], doctors disclosed as many details as they could, at the risk of embarrassing themselves and complicating their legal position . . . . In Baltimore in the past few weeks, Hopkins leaders initially chose to reveal little, at the risk of appearing to have something to hide." Eric Siegel and Diana K. Sugg, "Management of Crisis Key to Public Trust," *The Baltimore Sun*, June 24, 2001.

5. Aside from the obvious use of the label "monster study" as a pejorative to besmirch the reputations of the researcher and her supervisor, it is not otherwise totally clear what "monster study" is intended to convey. Is it that the researcher was a "monster" ("a cruel, wicked and inhuman person")? Is it that the study *produced* "monsters" ("a grossly malformed and usually nonviable fetus")? That the study actually made the subjects stronger ("someone or something that is abnormally large and powerful")? Certainly those who so describe the study do not mean to suggest that the study was a big hit in speech communication research, as in "a monster hit at the box office." (Quoted definitions from http://dictionary.com) Whichever of these meanings is intended by the use of "monster study" it is so totally devoid of factual basis as to leave it as little more than a purposeful attack on reputation.

6. The president of the Stuttering Foundation of America has also noted, "In the 60 intervening years, no other researcher [than Mary

Tudor] has demonstrated that labeling someone a stutterer or criticizing his speech alone leads to the development of stuttering." Jane Fraser, *The Fresno Bee*, July 10, 2001, p. B6.

7. "Inasmuch as there is willingness to recognize differences in standards that existed 60 years ago, the remaining major concern in the case of the Tudor study is whether or not the experimenter and her mentor intended to cause harm by turning normally speaking children into children who stutter. Our review of the study reveals no such apparent intent. The study investigated whether the level of disfluency could be changed as a result of labeling. It was not to create stutterers. Even if there was an unstated goal to increase disfluency to a level perceived as stuttered speech, there is no indication that Tudor or Johnson believed that, if successful, this would make the children chronic stutterers. This, in our opinion is a critical point in judging the ethics of those involved in the conduct of the study."

They conclude, "Our assessment of the ethical issues suggests that the study should be viewed within the common standards of the period, that there is no evidence of intent to harm, and that the objective of increasing disfluent speech should not be confused with instilling chronic stuttering in normally fluent children." (Ambrose & Yairi, 2002, p. 201)

8. The World Health Organization (WHO) is involved in evaluating the ethics of a number of aspects of medical care in developing countries. U.S. pharmaceutical companies have sometimes sold drugs in developing countries that have been rejected by the FDA for sale in the United States. Among the WHO's concerns are the ethical issues raised by the use of human subjects from developing countries in studies conducted by corporations and their researchers from the developed world. Concern for human subjects research ethics when the subjects are Americans tend to evaporate beyond our borders. As one author has put it, researchers are "changing their ethics 'at the customs desk.'" Paul M. McNeill (1998), "Should Research Ethics Change at the Border?" *The Medical Journal of Australia, 169,* 509–510, http://www.mja.com.au/public/issues/nov16/mcneill/mcneill.html

The WHO has an ethics page on the Web, http://www.who.int/ethics/en. One of its publications refers to "current ethical controversies as experienced in Argentina, Brazil, Canada, Colombia, Chile, Spain, the United States, Mexico and Peru."

The Centers for Disease Control and Prevention has a "Human Subjects Research" page (http://www.cdc.gov/od/ads/hsr2.htm) and provides the text of the Council for International Organizations of Medical Sciences (CIOMS), "International Guidelines for Ethical Review of Epidemiological Studies" (Geneva, 1991), http://www.cdc.gov/od/ads/intlgui3.htm

In March 2000, the *New England Journal of Medicine* reported a study reminiscent of Tuskegee (discussed in section II. D. 1., in the text) done by researchers from no less prestigious a research institution than Johns Hopkins. In the Rakai region of Uganda they monitored 415 couples of whom only one partner was infected with HIV. The researchers did not inform the AIDS-free partners. Thirty months later 90 of the formerly healthy spouses had become infected. The journal's editor charged that the study was unethical by U.S. standards. "Ethics of Medical Research in the Third World," *AllAfrica Global Media*, February 2, 2001, http://allafrica.com/stories/200102020128.html (subscription required). Five people died in a South African clinical trial of anti-AIDS drugs at the Kalafong hospital where participants "claimed they were ill-informed about their rights when they signed consent forms." Ibid.

Paul M. McNeill, cited above, reports that as a result of providing HIV-infected mothers with placebos as a part of studies in Thailand, Africa, and the Caribbean, their children were unnecessarily, and deliberately, permitted to develop AIDS.

9. That supersensitivity about human subject research ethics is both preventing research that needs to be done, and producing unfair moral judgments about that which has gone before, is supported by a couple of articles: Christopher Shea, "Don't Talk to the Humans," *Linquafranca*, 10(6), September 2000, and John R. Stanley, "Ethical Accusations: The Loss of Common Sense," *Archives of Dermatology*, 136(2), 268–269, February 2000, http://archderm.ama-assn.org/cgi/content/extract/136/2/268-a (extract only with link to subscription-based full text).

Shea discusses examples of IRBs interfering with research in anthropology, history, journalism, public policy (researchers' interviews with government officials), and urban ethnography. He cites the case of a history Ph.D. candidate who also works as a newspaper editor. "So during the day, when he's working on his dissertation, he is supposed to get permission from an IRB before he talks to a retired governor or columnist. . . . At night, he can call up anyone he wants and grill them."

Shea draws a stark contrast between the punctilious attention given by some to relatively harmless practices on the one hand (what he characterizes as the ethical equivalent of "run[ning] a red light on a deserted street at 3:00 AM."), and the somewhat less attention paid to much more serious ongoing ethical violations:

> You would not get the impression that human-subject committees are overly aggressive from reading the newspapers. In September 1999 a young man died while undergoing experimental gene therapy at the University of Pennsylvania, and his father subsequently claimed that no one had fully explained the risks involved in the treatment. Since the fall of 1998 the National Institutes of Health (NIH) have shut down research programs at eight institutions, including Duke University Medical Center, the University of Illinois at Chicago, and Virginia Commonwealth University. The NIH cited violations that ranged from inadequate record-keeping to a failure to review projects that should have been vetted.

One of the WHO ethics publications asserts that there is, "a growing perception that research involving human subjects is beneficial rather than threatening and that vulnerable groups, such as women, children, the elderly, and prisoners, should not be deprived arbitrarily of the opportunity to benefit from investigational drugs, vaccines or devices."

10. Much of the research regarding studies described in this section came from the Department of Energy's Advisory Committee on Human Radiation Experiments Report, DOE Openness: Human Radiation Experiments, http://tis.eh.doe.gov/ohre/roadmap/achre/ The Committee was established by the President in 1994. See especially "Part I. Ethics of Human Subjects Research: A Historical Perspective," http://tis.eh.doe.gov/ohre/roadmap/achre/overpt1.html

The U.S. Department of Health and Human Services' Office for Human Research Protections is a prime site for links to many of the basic documents both historical and current, http://www.hhs.gov/ohrp/ One of its pages provides links to educational material for researchers about human subjects ethics, http://www.hhs.gov/ohrp/education/index.html#materials

The Virginia Commonwealth University's site, "Ethics of Research Involving Human Participation," contains useful links: http://www.vcu.edu/hasweb/psy/faculty/fors/ethics.htm Professor Lawrence M. Hinman at the University of San Diego maintains an "Ethics Update" site, http://ethics.acusd.edu/

The National Library of Medicine's "Current Bibliographies in Medicine" series includes 5000 references in "Ethical Issues in Research Involving Human Participants," Current Bibliographies in Medicine 99–3, http://www.nlm.nih.gov/pubs/cbm/hum_exp.html The Introduction notes the significance of the President's 1997 apology to the

survivors of the Tuskegee Syphilis study and the reforms that followed. It says, "Contemporary safeguards such as [IRBs] are important, but by themselves are insufficient. Educating researchers and the
public about research ethics is critical for the full protection of research
participants." This bibliography is itself a consequence of that finding,
and the work of the Bioethics Education Materials and Resources Sub-
committee of the National Bioethics Advisory Commission.

11. The Nuremberg Code (1948) is a basic document available from
numerous sources and Web sites. One is, "Nuremberg Code: Directives
for Human Experimentation," Trials of War Criminals before the
Nuremberg Military Tribunals under Control Council Law No. 10, Vol.
2, pp. 181–182. Washington, DC: U.S. Government Printing Office, 1949,
http://ohsr.od.nih.gov/nuremberg.php3

12. World Medical Association, "World Medical Association Declaration of Helsinki Ethical Principles for Medical Research Involving
Human Subjects" ("Declaration of Helsinki") (Adopted by the 18th
World Medical Assembly, Helsinki, Finland, June 1964, and amended
by the 29th World Medical Assembly, Tokyo, Japan, October, 1975, 35th
World Medical Assembly, Venice, Italy, October 1983, 41st World Medical Assembly, Hong Kong, September 1989, 48th WMA General
Assembly, Somerset West, Republic of South Africa, October 1996, and
the 52nd WMA General Assembly, Edinburgh, Scotland, October 2000),
http://www.nihtraining.com/ohsrsite/guidelines/helsinki.html

And see Glen Drew, "Side-by-Side Comparison of 1996 and 2000 Declaration of Helsinki," http://www.hhs.gov/ohrp/nhrpac/mtg12-00/
h1996-2000.pdf

13. See, for example., NIH, Office of Human Subjects Research,
"Criteria for Institutional Review Board (IRB) Approval of Research
Involving Human Subjects," http://www.nihtraining.com/ohsrsite/
info/sheet3.html Criterion 2 provides, "An IRB may approve research
only after it has determined that all of the following requirements are
satisfied: . . . (b) Risks to subjects are reasonable relative to (1) anticipated benefits, if any, to subjects, and (2) the importance of the knowledge that may reasonably be expected to result."

14. This common defensive, and seemingly uncaring, reaction
continues to this day. Following the death of a subject during a 2001
Johns Hopkins study there was an expression of considerable outrage
by Johns Hopkins' doctors over the government's closing down their
research ("unwarranted, unnecessary, paralyzing and precipitous").

There was after all, they pointed out, only one dead subject. You would think it was they who were the victims rather than their dead human subject and her family members.

Nor was concern about loss of funding limited to Hopkins. The University of Iowa contributed to a local news story by Jim Jacobson, headlined "UI Funding Unaffected by Halt in Johns Hopkins Cancer Study," *Iowa City Gazette*, July 21, 2001, p. 1. Apparently Hopkins, rather than the government, subcontracts to the university $700,000 a year for one study and $11,000 for another. Iowa City residents were no doubt reassured to learn that the local research "likely will not be affected." There was no mention of the death, nor of expressions of concern by university administrators.

15. Even *Mercury News* reporter Jim Dyer later acknowledged, during an NPR interview, that "[Johnson] went to the . . . place that the University of Iowa . . . had used for several studies and research projects, and received permission . . . for this particular project." NPR, "Weekly Edition," June 23, 2001. He wrote, "In fact, in its 1936 biennial report, the Iowa State Board of Control, which oversaw all state institutions, openly encouraged and reported on cooperation with the University of Iowa in conducting research using children in various institutions." Jim Dyer, "Ethics and Orphans: The 'Monster Study,'" *San Jose Mercury News*, June 11, 2001. And see Colleen Krantz, "Orphans Targeted for Tests," *Des Moines Register*, July 9, 2001, p. 1. James Holmes, superintendent of the institution during the 1950s and 1960s has said of the Tudor study, "The state must have known about it" (Dyer, above).

16. References to the full text of the NASA standards, and their historical evolution, are a part of the Advisory Committee on Human Radiation Experiments Report; see Part I, Chapter 3, NASA Policy, http://www.eh.doe.gov/ohre/roadmap/achre/chap3_3.html

17. "The history of psychology . . . is studded with experiments whose designers gave too little thought to the well-being of their subjects . . . . [I]n the early 1960s the young Theodore Kaczynski—the future Unabomber—was among a group of Harvard students garlanded with electrodes and confronted by skilled lawyers who ridiculed and demolished what the students avowed were their most deeply held beliefs. No one explained the experiment in advance, the psychologists wanted to see how the students would handle the stress." Christopher Shea, "Don't Talk to the Humans: The Crackdown on Social Science Research," *Linguafranca*, *10*(6), September 2000. For additional references see, Nicholas Johnson, "Psychology's Special Problems," in "Cites, Sites, Sources and Notes," linked from http://www.nicholasjohnson.org

18. Even Tudor ethics critic Jim Dyer expressly acknowledges, "In the autumn of 1938, Johnson received permission from orphanage officials to begin his experiment." Jim Dyer, "Ethics and Orphans: The 'Monster Study,'" *San Jose Mercury News*, June 10, 2001. He continues, "The university had already conducted numerous research projects . . . there, among them a decades-long study to see if developmental retardation would be more common among children who remained in the overcrowded and unstimulating orphanage than among children placed in a special new preschool."

19. Retired Marquette speech pathology professor Bill Trotter agrees: "I know Wendell Johnson was an extremely ethical and moral person, and if something happened to those children it was because of something he did not foresee." Jim Dyer, "Ethics and Orphans: the 'Monster Study,'" *San Jose Mercury News*, June 11, 2001.

20. For any readers totally unaware of the reputation of Dr. Wendell Johnson for ethical, kindly and thoughtful behavior toward others, a few quotes and a Web site link may provide some insight.

Shortly after the *Mercury News* articles the former director of the Indiana University Speech, Language and Hearing Clinics wrote, "Johnson . . . completed a formidable body of scientific research that gave hope to millions. Johnson was a remarkable personality who got along well with everyone. His stuttering clients, their families, university students, etc. all loved him. He was such a kind man. There was nothing that he would ever have done intentionally to harm anyone." Robert L. Milisen, "Johnson Was a Great Man," *Iowa City Press-Citizen*, June 27, 2001, p. 11A.

Former colleague Dr. D. C. Spriestersbach told Jim Dyer, "Wendell Johnson was a most revered and universally loved man." Jim Dyer, "Ethics and Orphans: The 'Monster Study,'" *San Jose Mercury News*, June 11, 2001.

Five speech pathologists wrote, "Recently have come comparisons of Dr. Wendell Johnson to Timothy McVeigh and Adolf Hitler. This has made us so angry. Johnson has no similarities to such individuals. He was a fine man, dedicated to helping solve the problems of stuttering, not only in the United States but also in the world. All that has been accomplished in this emotion-laden journalism is the trashing of a well-earned reputation of one of the most decent men who ever lived."

Judith Knabe, Peggy Gingerich, Nancy Fesenmeyer, Jill Lorack, and Becky Hubbard, "Wendell Johnson was a Fine Man: Judge Him in Light of the Times," *Iowa City Gazette*, July 5, 2001, p. 7A.

Even while issuing the University's apology to surviving subjects of the Tudor study, the University's Vice President for Research, David Skorton, who was very critical of the study's ethics, added, "In no way does this statement denigrate Wendell Johnson's very important and contributory career. He was a huge, positive factor in the field of speech pathology and in the lives of many, many patients with speech disorders." Kathryn Ratliff, "UI Apologizes for Research on Stuttering," *Iowa City Press-Citizen*, June 14, 2001, p. 1A.

A former student and colleague wrote of him after his death, "He was much beloved, even by those in Iowa City who knew little of his international recognition and awards. To them he was a neighbor, a great public speaker, teller of stories, composer of songs and limericks, personal counselor and active member of civic organizations. When he died, in addition to the stories in national news magazines and newspapers, the family was flooded with thousands of letters from individuals around the world, formerly unknown to them, who had been touched in some way by his life and love of humankind." Dean Williams, "Remembering Wendell Johnson," *Et cetera*, Winter 1992–93, p. 433, reprinted from the *Daily Iowan*, May 4, 1992.

> The man I knew seemed exceedingly gentle and incapable of angering. His disposition had a very calming effect in otherwise trying times . . . . A few days before he died in August 1965, I received a very long letter with remarks on his health status, general philosophizing, and the wish that he could be 50 white rats so his physicians could do the kind of research on his condition that could provide some answers, a typically Johnsonian approach to life. . . . To sum up the Johnson I knew, my best memories are of a pleasant, jovial, dedicated man whose love of life and of people was evidenced in his every act. (Joseph L. Stewart, "Wendell Johnson: A Memoir," *Et cetera*, Winter 1992–1993, p. 424.)

See generally, "Wendell A. L. Johnson Memorial Home Page." Available as a link from: http://www.nicholasjohnson.org

21. See also Dorothy Moeller, *Speech Pathology and Audiology: Iowa Origins of a Discipline* (Iowa City: University of Iowa, 1975), pp. 61–62.

22. "As you can see, the woman 'featured' in Dyer's articles actually got more fluent over the four months." Dr. Robert W. Quesal, E-mail to author, June 21, 2001, with accompanying supporting analysis of the Tudor study data.

23. Dr. Wendell Johnson's masters thesis, *Because I Stutter* (Appleton, 1930), was one of the very few masters theses to be commercially published. Although out of print, it is available on the Web as a link from http://www.nicholasjohnson.org/wjohnson

24. The masters thesis is a very thin document consisting of no more than a handful of pages of commentary and conclusions along with a reproduction of the data. Moreover, twenty-first century critics of the study argue that the data it contains simply do not support its few conclusions. Few masters theses in any field are likely to receive much attention and subsequent citation, so it is not remarkable that the Tudor study did not. However, in this case it is at least possible that an additional reason for the little attention it received over the years is that earlier researchers saw in it the same flaws seen by its critics a half-century later. In any event, given that it was cataloged in the University of Iowa Library, as accessible as any other masters thesis over the years, and checked out many times, this seems a much more probable explanation than that it was "suppressed."

25. Standards change over time with regard to many aspects of human behavior. Language widely used without formal objection at one time, say, the way some men talked about women during the 1950s, may become the basis for everything from social shunning to law suits for sexual harassment decades later.

The writer was a human subject in a University of Iowa clinical trial of a new drug. It is apparently standard practice to require human subjects, who are taking at least some risk for no pay in a project from which everyone else is profiting, to sign a couple of waivers. One absolves the institution not only from any liability for harm, but even liability for negligence. The other seems especially uncaring. The testing institution, a major research hospital, expressly leaves human subjects harmed by the study entirely on their own in their search, and ability to pay, for restorative medical care. Is this ethical? Under 2001 standards apparently it is. Will there be another view of the matter in the future? One would hope so. And, if so, will moral outrage then be expressed regarding those who utilized such overreaching waiver language today? One would hope not.

By mid-twenty-first century a majority of the world's population may conclude that today's animal rights activists were right all along. Those not vegetarians in 2001 may find their eating habits subsequently described as "barbaric" some 62 years later because of their earlier willingness to slaughter animals and eat their flesh. They may even become named defendants in mock trials for their participation in this animal genocide. PETA (People for the Ethical Treatment of Animals) has for years objected to the use of animals in research, http://www.pe ta.org and see especially, "Cruel Science," http://www.peta.org/cmp/ sci.html and "Stop Animal Tests," http://www.stopanimal tests.com

The citizens of many countries already regard Americans as barbarians because we continue the death penalty, a practice they believe violates the United Nation's Universal Declaration of Human Rights (1948), http://www.un.orgt/Overview/rights.html, as President George W. Bush discovered during his 2001 European trip.

Those who are insistent on applying the standards of their day to the human subjects research of others in the 1920s and 1930s might at least want to consider the consequences of doing so. To apply early twenty-first century standards to early twentieth century research will mean that, for the next few years, professional societies, research universities, and other institutions will be issuing apologies to the thousands of experimental subjects of that time, if not writing checks for billions of dollars as well. Indeed, one journalist has already seriously suggested they should be doing just that. John Carlson, "U of I, State Owe Yesteryear's Orphans the Whole Truth," *Des Moines Register*, June 17, 2001, p. 1B.

26. Although best known as a speech pathologist, Dr. Wendell Johnson was also one of the founders of the International Society for General Semantics. His book, *People in Quandaries*, first published in 1946, was still available in 2001.

27. It was December 2002 before the State of Oregon first acknowledged that its program of forced sterilization was no longer acceptable. From 1917 through 1983 over 2500 Oregonians, "girls in reform school, people in mental institutions and poor women selected by welfare workers," were sterilized. AP, "Ore. Gov. Apologizes for Sterilization," December 2, 2002.

28. Gina Kolata, "U.S. Suspends Human Research at Johns Hopkins After a Death," *The New York Times*, July 20, 2001.

The most detailed reporting regarding the Johns Hopkins controversy was, not surprisingly, in *The Baltimore Sun*.

Jonathan Bor and Tom Pelton, "Hopkins Study Was Exempt from FDA; Asthma Project Tested Function of Lungs, Wasn't a Drug Trial," *The Baltimore Sun*, June 22, 2001.

Jonathan Bor, "Hopkins Panel to Study Death of Volunteer," *The Baltimore Sun*, June 23, 2001.

Eric Siegel and Diana K. Sugg, "Management of Crisis Key to Public Trust," *The Baltimore Sun*, June 24, 2001.

Douglas M. Birch and Gary Cohn, "The Changing Creed of Hopkins Science; What Once Was Heresy Is Now the Mission: A Partnership with Business to Advance Research," *The Baltimore Sun*, June 25, 2001.

Editorial, "Death at Research Center; Hopkins Study: Volunteer's Death Raises Questions About Protection, Role of Human Research Subjects," *The Baltimore Sun*, July 1, 2001.

Editorial, "Of Profits and Patients; Medical Research: Academic Institutions Face Huge Conflicts of Interest as They Pursue Business Ties," *The Baltimore Sun*, July 2, 2001.

Tom Pelton, "Asthma Study Violated Safety Rules, FDA Says; Hopkins Experiment Ended with Death of Volunteer, 24," *The Baltimore Sun*, July 3, 2001.

Tom Pelton, "Respected Doctors Confront a Tragedy; Experiment: With a Research Subject's Death, Two Distinguished Scientists Confront What Colleagues Say Is the Worst Imaginable Outcome," *The Baltimore Sun*, July 8, 2001.

Editorial, "An Unnecessary Death; Hopkins Study: Tighter Controls on Human Research Projects Needed; Institution's Inquiry Finds Faults," *The Baltimore Sun*, July 18, 2001.

Jonathan Bor and Tom Pelton, "U.S. Halts Hopkins Research; Most Experiments on Human Subjects Ordered Suspended; Federal Funding Withheld; Oversight Agency Decries Safety Lapses in Volunteer's Death," *The Baltimore Sun*, July 20, 2001.

Michael Stroh, "Shutdowns Have Wide Effect on Programs; Cutting-edge Treatments Become Unavailable; Funding, Name Damaged," *The Baltimore Sun*, July 20, 2001.

"Hopkins Calls Federal Agency's Action 'Precipitous,'" *The Baltimore Sun*, July 20, 2001.

Editorial, "Protecting Humans in Research; Hopkins Shutdown: Government Is Right to Be Concerned, but Wrong to Punish Researchers so Harshly," *The Baltimore Sun*, July 21, 2001.

Diana K. Sugg, "Despite Suspension, Hopkins Researchers Continue Vital Tests; Doctors, Nurses Rush to Reassure Patients, Appeal Research Bans," *The Baltimore Sun*, July 21, 2001.

Tom Pelton and Jonathan Bor, "Hopkins Vows to Improve Research Safety; Changes Outlined in Letter School Sent to Federal Agency; 'It's Been Utter Confusion;' Lifting of Suspension Sought by Next Week," *The Baltimore Sun*, July 21, 2001.

29. See also, "UI Apologizes for Stuttering Study," *San Jose Mercury News*, June 14, 2001; "University Apologizes for '39 Experiment," *Chicago Tribune*, June 14, 2001, p. 19. University of Iowa President Mary

Sue Coleman was quoted as saying, "There's no way I can condone that kind of research." Jim Jacobson, "UI Denounces Experiment," *Iowa City Gazette*, June 13, 2001, p. 1A. Richard Hurtig, Chair of the UI Department of Speech Pathology and Audiology was quoted as saying that "this is not the kind of study anyone today would even think of proposing or would an institutional review board authorize." Kathryn A. Ratliff, "UI Stuttering Study Doubted," *Iowa City Press-Citizen*, June 12, 2001, pp. 1, 7.

30. James Dyer, "The Twisted Experiment of Dr. Wendell Johnson," *The Iowa City Mercury*, April 1992, p. 1. Franklin Silverman reported on the Tudor study as early as 1988 in the *Journal of Fluency Disorders*. It was also the subject of a novel by Jerry Halvorson in 1999.

31. The suggestion that today's research institutions and individuals possess a moral superiority to their predecessors, that there are standards in place today to prevent any possibility of the problems of earlier times, is a triumph of arrogance over experience. The abuses detailed in the DHHS Office of Inspector General's report, "Protecting Human Research Subjects," were published as recently as April 2000. It is available online in pdf format, http://www.oig.hhs.gov/oei/reports/oei-01-97-00197.pdf

The NIH requirement of "education on the protection of human research participants for all investigations" was established even later, in October 2000. One institutional response has been a simple online summary presentation of some highlights that researchers are required to scan. An example is the University of Michigan's "Protection of Human Research Subjects Computer-Based Training for Researchers." A comparable online training program is The National Cancer Institute, "Human Participant Protections Education for Research Teams," http://cme.cancer.gov/clinicaltrials/learning/humanparticipant -protections.asp (requires free online registration). Stanford University offers a similar "Use of Human Subjects in Research: History" tutorial module, http://www.stanford.edu/department/DoR/hs/History/h is01.html

32. Less than one week after the Johns Hopkins revelations the *Des Moines* [Iowa] *Register* headlined on page one: "U of I Faces Probe Over Research." The story noted that, among other things, "the issues raised . . . focus on internal review boards that sometimes rushed approval of changes in experiment guidelines and did not document procedures in enough detail." Colleen Krantz, "U of I Faces Probe Over Research," *Des Moines Sunday Register*, July 22, 2001, p. 1.

A letter to the university in 1999 from the Food and Drug Administration referred to its reviews at the university in 1992, 1995, and 1998. Each of those reviews involved violations that "are of particular importance because many of them have been observed during past inspections where corrections were promised by your institution but not implemented." According to the news story, an FDA spokesperson said it is "fairly rare to see issues remain unresolved after several visits, as inspectors suggested was the case at the University of Iowa."

A spokesperson for the university tried to minimize, even trivialize, the violations as "minor administrative details." Said another, "the more complex the research the greater the likelihood there are some failures because we are, after all, all human." Thus was it revealed that the standard of at least some educational administrators is to be forgiving of their own ethical and legal errors, but morally outraged by those of their predecessors.

The same University spokesperson who joined in the chorus of moral outrage, saying that the Tudor study was "unfortunate and indefensible," was later quoted in a local paper's follow-up on the *Register* exposé of the University's own failings. The *Register* reported that, "The university calls into question both the headline and its [the story's] placement as Sunday's leading story," while acknowledging that the story itself was "mostly accurate if read in its entirety."

The University of Iowa's continuing tenacious campaign against the *Des Moines Register's* headline and placement was represented in a letter to the editor with a headline presumably finally thought acceptable, David Skorton, "No Action Pending Regarding U of I Research," Opinion, *Des Moines Register*, August 5, 2001, p. 9A.

The contrast between this protest by the University over the headline and placement of a story it concedes was "balanced and mostly accurate," and its response to the media's unethical and broadside attacks on the 1939 Tudor study are striking. In the latter case it not only failed to protest *anything* about the stories, whether content, headlines, or placement, it actually joined in the moral castigation of its own former faculty member.

There was, of course, no reference to how "unfortunate and indefensible" it is that clear governmental standards have not been complied with in spite of repeated government investigations and university assurances of correction. See generally, George Pappas, "Gov't Probe of UI Research 'Minor,'" *The Daily Iowan*, July 23, 2001, p. 1; George Pappas, "UI Fires Back at Register's Headline," *The Daily Iowan*, July 24, 2001, p. 1; Ryan Foley, "'Monster Study' Reporter Under Fire," *The Daily Iowan*, July 26, 2001, p. 1.

33. One of many possible consequences of such a hurried rush to public relations offensive is its impact on litigation. With potential plaintiffs waiting in the wings, to launch a gratuitous assault on a former faculty member as someone who supervised "a study that should [n]ever be considered defensible in any era," however much thought to be potentially useful in the public relations short run, is a somewhat reckless gamble with a state university's resources.

34. As one speech pathologist has noted, "Even more startling than the [Dyer] article itself was its front-page placement and space allotment, this for an article appearing to provide no useful information whatsoever to the public. . . . How much more useful would an article about stuttering problems have been if readers had instead been informed of resources. . . . As a speech pathologist, I am particularly disheartened that the opportunity to help people prevent and treat stuttering problems was squandered in what seems to be efforts to engage in sensationalism, for what purpose or purposes one can only speculate." Ellen-Marie Silverman, "Paper Missed Chance to Better Inform Readers," *Milwaukee Journal Sentinel*, June 18, 2001, p. 10A.

35. See, for example, Dorothy Moeller, *Speech Pathology and Audiology: Iowa Origins of a Discipline* (Iowa City: University of Iowa, 1975); Wendell Johnson, *Because I Stutter* (New York: Appleton, 1930); Wendell Johnson, *People in Quandaries* (New York: Harper & Brothers, 1946); Wendell Johnson (Ed.), *Stuttering in Children and Adults* (Minneapolis: University of Minnesota Press, 1955); Wendell Johnson (Ed.), *The Onset of Stuttering: Research Findings and Implications* (Minneapolis: University of Minnesota Press, 1959).

36. There are numerous ethical issues in human subjects research truly deserving of academic reflection and public education by journalists. Here is but one example.

An April 2000 report of the DHHS Office of Inspector General, "Protecting Human Research Subjects," notes a great many "disturbing inadequacies." One, it says, is that "The increased commercialization of research and the growing importance of research revenues for institutions heightens the potential for conflicts of interest in clinical research."

On August 5, 2001, the *Washington Post* reported that overreaching by pharmaceutical companies was so bad that "editors at the world's most prominent medical journals, alarmed that drug companies are exercising too much control over research results, have agreed to adopt a uniform policy that reserves the right to refuse to publish drug company-sponsored studies. . . . " Susan Okie, "A Stand for Scientific Independence: Medical Journals Aim to Curtail Drug Companies' Influence," *Washington Post*, August 5, 2001, p. A1. (The story was reported in Iowa City as, "Journals Adopt New Policy: Editors Aim to Clip Drug Companies' Influence," *Iowa City Press-Citizen*, August 5, 2001, p. 1A, and "Medical Journals Battle Drug Firms' Grip on Research," *Iowa City Gazette*, August 5, 2001, p. 3A.)

The author quotes "several observers of biomedical studies who have become alarmed about the influence of the drug industry on the integrity of medical research." A University of California professor of clinical pharmacy is quoted as saying that if negative results are published "you can still get pressure put on you for fear that you won't get any future funding." Companies not only control access to data, but may even control who writes the papers, or ghost writes them for the academics who "are too busy to take all the time needed to create the publication." She cites examples in which reports of side effects, no benefits, or cheaper alternatives have led to blocked publication or even lawsuits.

One would think the significance of an ethical issue of this magnitude would be worth at least as much media attention as a masters thesis from 1939.

37. Compare Greg Mitchell, "Reporters Trail Badly (Again) in Annual Poll on Honesty and Ethics," Editor and Publisher, December 7, 2004 ("Once again, newspaper reporters score poorly in the annual Gallup Poll . . . on 'honesty and ethical standards' in various professions . . . lower than bankers, auto mechanics, elected officials, and nursing-home operators"), http://www.editorandpublisher.com/ eandp/news/article_display.jsp?vnu_content_id=1000732750 with Michelle Z. Spielman, "U.S. Journalists Get High Marks on Ethics, Study Finds; LSU and University of Missouri professors analyze the 'moral minds' of journalists and advertisers," *LSU's Biweekly Newsletter for Faculty & Staff*, 21(12), February 25, 2005, http://www.lsu.edu/lsu-today/050225/pageone.html , and Kelly McBride, "Journalists: More

Ethical than People Realize?," Poynteronline, December 17, 2004, http://
www.poynter.org/content/content_print.asp?id=75962&custom=

38. "As you can see, the woman 'featured' in Dyer's articles actu-
ally got more fluent over the four months." Dr. Robert W. Quesal,
E-mail to author, June 21, 2001, with accompanying analysis of the
Tudor study data.

39. The *Mercury News* ethics policy, violated by the journalist,
provides:

> Under ordinary circumstances, reporters or photographers ought to
> identify themselves to news sources. There might be times, however,
> when circumstances will dictate not identifying ourselves. Only the
> Executive Editor or Editor may approve such exceptions. (*Mercury
> News* Ethics Policy, September 21, 2004, http://www.grandforks.com/
> mld/mercurynews/contact_us/about/9723906.htm)

To which the Executive Editor added in his editorial, "I didn't." David
Yarnold, "Setting the Record Straight," *The San Jose Mercury News*, July
25, 2001.

40. The quote is from a promotional, public relations release from
Patty Wise, the *Mercury News'* Public Relations Manager, distributed
nationally by the PR Newswire Association, "to medical, family and
features editors," June 8, 2001. It made both stories available to other
papers prior to their publication in the *Mercury News*, thus ensuring the
re-enforcing impact of the national media blitz.

41. The false claim that the study was "revealed for the first time"
in the *Mercury News'* stories of 2001 is particularly ironic and unethical
given that the stories' author, Jim Dyer, was *himself* one of those who
wrote about it earlier in the *Iowa City Mercury*. James Dyer, "The
Twisted Experiment of Dr. Wendell Johnson," *The Iowa City Mercury*,
April 1992, p. 1. Franklin Silverman reported on the Tudor study as
early as 1988 in the *Journal of Fluency Disorders*. Franklin Silverman,
"The monster study," *Journal of Fluency Disorders*, 13, 225–231 (1988).
(For a different view of the Tudor study and its media coverage from
the Silverman family see the quote from Ellen-Marie Silverman, "Paper
Missed Chance to Better Inform Readers," *Milwaukee Journal Sentinel*,
June 18, 2001, p. 10A, note 34, above.) The study was also the subject of
a novel by Jerry Halvorson in 1999, Jerry Halvorson, *Abandoned: Now
Stutter My Orphan* (1999) (with foreword by Franklin Silverman).

American Speech-Language-Hearing Association Code of Ethics[*]

Last Revised January 1, 2003

Preamble

The preservation of the highest standards of integrity and ethical principles is vital to the responsible discharge of obligations by speech-language pathologists, audiologists, and speech, language, and hearing scientists. This Code of Ethics sets forth the fundamental principles and rules considered essential to this purpose.

Every individual who is (a) a member of the American Speech-Language-Hearing Association, whether certified or not, (b) a nonmember holding the Certificate of Clinical Competence from the Association, (c) an applicant for membership or certification, or (d) a Clinical Fellow seeking to fulfill standards for certification shall abide by this Code of Ethics.

Any violation of the spirit and purpose of this Code shall be considered unethical. Failure to specify any particular responsibility or practice in this Code of Ethics shall not be construed as denial of the existence of such responsibilities or practices.

The fundamentals of ethical conduct are described by Principles of Ethics and by Rules of Ethics as they relate to the conduct of research and scholarly activities and responsibility to persons

*Reprinted by permission from American-Speech-Language-Hearing Association. Code of ethics (revised 2003). *ASHA Supplement, 23*, pp. 13–15. Copyright 2003 by American Speech-Language-Hearing Association.

served, the public, and speech-language pathologists, audiologists, and speech, language, and hearing scientists.

Principles of Ethics, aspirational and inspirational in nature, form the underlying moral basis for the Code of Ethics. Individuals shall observe these principles as affirmative obligations under all conditions of professional activity.

Rules of Ethics are specific statements of minimally acceptable professional conduct or of prohibitions and are applicable to all individuals.

Principle of Ethics I

Individuals shall honor their responsibility to hold paramount the welfare of persons they serve professionally or participants in research and scholarly activities and shall treat animals involved in research in a humane manner.

Rules of Ethics

A. Individuals shall provide all services competently.

B. Individuals shall use every resource, including referral when appropriate, to ensure that high-quality service is provided.

C. Individuals shall not discriminate in the delivery of professional services or the conduct of research and scholarly activities on the basis of race or ethnicity, gender, age, religion, national origin, sexual orientation, or disability.

D. Individuals shall not misrepresent the credentials of assistants, technicians, or support personnel and shall inform those they serve professionally of the name and professional credentials of persons providing services.

E. Individuals who hold the Certificates of Clinical Competence shall not delegate tasks that require the unique skills, knowledge, and judgment that are within the scope of their profession to assistants, technicians, support personnel, students, or any nonprofessionals over whom they have supervisory responsibility. An individual may delegate support services to assistants, technicians, support personnel, students, or any other persons only if those services are adequately supervised by an individual who holds the appropriate Certificate of Clinical Competence.

F. Individuals shall fully inform the persons they serve of the nature and possible effects of services rendered and products dispensed, and they shall inform participants in research about the possible effects of their participation in research conducted.

G. Individuals shall evaluate the effectiveness of services rendered and of products dispensed and shall provide services or dispense products only when benefit can reasonably be expected.

H. Individuals shall not guarantee the results of any treatment or procedure, directly or by implication; however, they may make a reasonable statement of prognosis.

I. Individuals shall not provide clinical services solely by correspondence.

J. Individuals may practice by telecommunication (for example, telehealth/e-health), where not prohibited by law.

K. Individuals shall adequately maintain and appropriately secure records of professional services rendered, research and scholarly activities conducted, and products dispensed and shall allow access to these records only when authorized or when required by law.

L. Individuals shall not reveal, without authorization, any professional or personal information about identified persons served professionally or identified participants involved in research and scholarly activities unless required by law to do so, or unless doing so is necessary to protect the welfare of the person or of the community or otherwise required by law.

M. Individuals shall not charge for services not rendered, nor shall they misrepresent services rendered, products dispensed, or research and scholarly activities conducted.

N. Individuals shall use persons in research or as subjects of teaching demonstrations only with their informed consent.

O. Individuals whose professional services are adversely affected by substance abuse or other health-related conditions shall seek professional assistance and, where appropriate, withdraw from the affected areas of practice.

Principle of Ethics II

Individuals shall honor their responsibility to achieve and maintain the highest level of professional competence.

Rules of Ethics

A. Individuals shall engage in the provision of clinical services only when they hold the appropriate Certificate of Clinical Competence or when they are in the certification process and are supervised by an individual who holds the appropriate Certificate of Clinical Competence.

B. Individuals shall engage in only those aspects of the professions that are within the scope of their competence, considering their level of education, training, and experience.

C. Individuals shall continue their professional development throughout their careers.

D. Individuals shall delegate the provision of clinical services only to: (1) persons who hold the appropriate Certificate of Clinical Competence; (2) persons in the education or certification process who are appropriately supervised by an individual who holds the appropriate Certificate of Clinical Competence; or (3) assistants, technicians, or support personnel who are adequately supervised by an individual who holds the appropriate Certificate of Clinical Competence.

E. Individuals shall not require or permit their professional staff to provide services or conduct research activities that exceed the staff member's competence, level of education, training, and experience.

F. Individuals shall ensure that all equipment used in the provision of services or to conduct research and scholarly activities is in proper working order and is properly calibrated.

Principle of Ethics III

Individuals shall honor their responsibility to the public by promoting public understanding of the professions, by supporting the development of services designed to fulfill the unmet needs of the public, and by providing accurate information in all communications involving any aspect of the professions, including dissemination of research findings and scholarly activities.

Rules of Ethics

A. Individuals shall not misrepresent their credentials, competence, education, training, experience, or scholarly or research contributions.

B. Individuals shall not participate in professional activities that constitute a conflict of interest.

C. Individuals shall refer those served professionally solely on the basis of the interest of those being referred and not on any personal financial interest.

D. Individuals shall not misrepresent diagnostic information, research, services rendered, or products dispensed; neither shall they engage in any scheme to defraud in connection with obtaining payment or reimbursement for such services or products.

E. Individuals' statements to the public shall provide accurate information about the nature and management of communication disorders, about the professions, about professional services, and about research and scholarly activities.

F. Individuals' statements to the public—advertising, announcing, and marketing their professional services, reporting research results, and promoting products—shall adhere to prevailing professional standards and shall not contain misrepresentations.

Principle of Ethics IV

Individuals shall honor their responsibilities to the professions and their relationships with colleagues, students, and members of allied professions. Individuals shall uphold the dignity and autonomy of the professions, maintain harmonious interprofessional and extraprofessional relationships, and accept the professions' self-imposed standards.

Rules of Ethics

A. Individuals shall prohibit anyone under their supervision from engaging in any practice that violates the Code of Ethics.

B. Individuals shall not engage in dishonesty, fraud, deceit, misrepresentation, sexual harrassment, or any other form of conduct that adversely reflects on the professions or on the individual's fitness to serve persons professionally.

C. Individuals shall not engage in sexual activities with clients or students over whom they exercise professional authority.

D. Individuals shall assign credit only to those who have contributed to a publication, presentation, or product. Credit shall be assigned in proportion to the contribution and only with the contributor's consent.

E. Individuals shall reference the source when using other persons' ideas, research, presentations, or products in written, oral, or any other media presentation or summary.

F. Individuals' statements to colleagues about professional services, research results, and products shall adhere to prevailing professional standards and shall contain no misrepresentations.

G. Individuals shall not provide professional services without exercising independent professional judgment, regardless of referral source or prescription.

H. Individuals shall not discriminate in their relationships with colleagues, students, and members of allied professions on the basis of race or ethnicity, gender, age, religion, national origin, sexual orientation, or disability.

I. Individuals who have reason to believe that the Code of Ethics has been violated shall inform the Board of Ethics.

J. Individuals shall comply fully with the policies of the Board of Ethics in its consideration and adjudication of complaints of violations of the Code of Ethics.

INDEX

A

Allen, Woody, xii
American Psychological Association
(APA), 77
ethics code, 84
American Speech-Language-Hearing
Association (ASHA), *See*
ASHA (American Speech-
Language-Hearing
Association)
APA (American Psychological
Association), *See* American
Psychological Association
(APA)
Aristotle, 13
ASHA (American Speech-Language-
Hearing Association)
accusation apology, xiii
Certificate of Clinical Competence
(CCC), 64
Code of Ethics, 63, 71, 73, 84
history of, 64–65
research participant issues, 95
and research/scholarship, 64–65
revised, 2003, 134
text, 201–207
ethical issues, current, 65–71
and ethics instruction, 62
Rules of Ethics, 207

Asimov, Isaac, xii
Assessment, 17–21
set theory model, 22–25
"A to Z" list (Van Riper), 14

B

Baltimore Sun exposé, 140, 184n4,
193–194n28
Because I Stutter (Johnson), 6, 192n23
Belmont Report, 86–88, 132–133, 153,
See also under Participants,
research
Bloodstein, Oliver, xv, 6, 7, 8, 11, 25
doctoral dissertation of, 32
retirement address, 124
stuttering reduction/absence, 32
and stuttering research, U. of Iowa
(c. 1939), 27–33
theories, 122–124
Byron, George Gordon (Lord), xii

C

CAPCSD (Council of Academic
Programs in
Communication Sciences
and Disorders), 72

210 ETHICS: A CASE STUDY

CCC (Certificate of Clinical Competence), ASHA, 64
Centers for Disease Control and Prevention, 185–186n8
Cicero, xi
City University of New York (CUNY) Graduate Center ethics instruction, 78–81
Cluttering, 118
Code of Ethics (ASHA), 63, 71, 73, 84
  history of, 64–65
  research participant issues, 95
  and research/scholarship, 64–65
  revised, 2003, 134
  text, 201–207
Coleridge, Samuel Taylor, xii
Common Rule regulations, 83–84
Communication sciences/disorders researcher decline, 134–135
Construct validity, 118–119
Continuity hypothesis (Bloodstein), 14
Council of Academic Programs in Communication Sciences and Disorders (CAPCSD), 72
CUNY (City University of New York) Graduate Center ethics instruction, 78–81

D

Diagnosis
  differential, 16–17
  and treatment, 21–22
Diagnosogenic theory, xi, xiii, 14
  alternative hypotheses, 118
  contemporary view, 58
  evidence for, 29
  genesis of, 8, 42
  as intervention underpinning, 10–11
  Johnson devotion to, 28
  as oversimplification, 14
  scope of, 43–44
  and Tudor study, 28, 38, 41, 43
  verification of, 28–29

Disfluency, *See also* Stuttering
  frequency, 19
  normal
    in preschoolers, 16
    and stuttering, 13–15, 33, 45–46
  prolongation duration, 19–20
  and stuttering, 44–45
  type, 18–19

E

Electromyography, 2, 98–101
Encyclopaedia Britannica article (Johnson), 12, 28
Ethics, *See also* Tudor study
  and AIDS, 154–155, 158, 166–168, 185–186n8
  atomic bomb testing, 148, 162
  Beecher report, 155
  changing over time, 63, 141, 144–155, 185n7, 192–193n25
  chimpanzee-to-human kidney transplant attempt, 150, 154
  coercion, 66–68
  Common Rule regulations, 83–84
  contemporary problems, 152
  current issues, 65–71
  in developing countries, 154–155, 158
  hepatitis infection of persons who were retarded, 150–151, 158
  informed consent, 55, 69–71, 88, 157–158
  instruction in, 71–73
    City University of New York (CUNY) Graduate Center, 78–81
    Mercy College, 76–78
    Molloy College, 74–76
    National Institutes of Health (NIH), 77–78, 80
  Johns Hopkins AIDS study, 140, 166–168, 185–186n8, 195–197n32
  and Johnson, Wendell, 27
  and judgment lapse, 33

O

Office of Human Research Protection
(OHRP), 89, 95
higher-risk approval, 90
The Onset of Stuttering (Johnson), 10,
28
OPRP (Office of Human Research
Protection), 89
Overview, 1–12, 35

P

Participants, research, *See also* Public
Law 93-348 (National
Research Act)
approval, higher-risk research, 90
autonomy, 87
background, 2
Belmont Report, 86–88, 132–133
beneficence, 87–88
justice, 88
respect, 87
benefit/harm balancing, 87–88, 89
children, 88, 89–91
advocates, 91
with communication disorders,
93–94
ethics, overall, 156
feral, 85
parents/guardians, 90–91
Part D (PL 93-348, 89–91
19th century, 84–85
cognitive-linguistic ability, 90
fairness, 88
history of protection, 84–91
informed consent, 55, 69–71, 88,
157–158
National Commission for the
Protection of Human
Subjects of Biomedical and
Behavioral Research, 86, 89
National Research Act (PL 93-348),
86, 89–91
Nazi human experiments, 85, 88

Participants, research *(continued)*
and parents/guardians, 90
and power differential, 87
Recommendations Guiding
Medical Doctors in
Biomedical Research
Involving Human Subjects,
86
selection criteria, nonscientific, 89
Tuskegee syphilis study, xiii, 86,
88, 147–148, 152–153, 162
wards of a
state/institution/agency, 91,
92, 156–157
Willowbrook Psychiatric Institute
(Long Island), 86
PFSP (Hollins Precision Fluency
Shaping Program), 105–110
Pharmaceutical research, 197–198n36
Physiological studies, stuttering
electromyographic research, 98–101
and Hollins Precision Fluency
Shaping Program (PFSP),
105–110
invasive technique, 98–101
minimally invasive techniques,
101–114
pretherapy patterns, 102–104
respiratory research, 101–104
tongue-to-other-articulators
measures, 110–114
and x-ray microbeam, 112
Plagiarism, 76, 80–81
Power of professor and research,
131–135
Precision Fluency Shaping Program
(PFSP), 105–110
Privacy, 55
*Professional Issues in Speech-Language
Pathology and Audiology*
(Lubinski & Frattali), 78
Professor, power of, and research,
131–135
*Publication Manual of the American
Psychological Association*
(APA), 77